100 Questions & Answers About Mesothelioma

Second Edition

Harvey I. Pass, MD
Professor of Cardiothoracic Surgery and Surgery
Director, Division of Thoracic Surgery and Thoracic Oncology
Department of Cardiothoracic Surgery
NYU School of Medicine and Clinical Cancer Center
New York, New York

Amy Metula, BSN, RN, MA, ANP-C
Quality Performance Manager
Weill Cornell Medical College
New York, NY

Susan Vento
Education Minnesota Field Staff
St. Paul, MN

JONES AND BARTLETT PUBLISHERS
Sudbury, Massachusetts
BOSTON   TORONTO   LONDON   SINGAPORE

World Headquarters

Jones and Bartlett
Publishers
40 Tall Pine Drive
Sudbury, MA 01776
978-443-5000
info@jbpub.com
www.jbpub.com

Jones and Bartlett
Publishers Canada
6339 Ormindale Way
Mississauga, Ontario L5V 1J2
CANADA

Jones and Bartlett
Publishers International
Barb House, Barb Mews
London W6 7PA
United Kingdom

Jones and Bartlett's books and products are available through most bookstores and online book-sellers. To contact Jones and Bartlett Publishers directly, call 800-832-0034, fax 978-443-8000, or visit our website www.jbpub.com.

Substantial discounts on bulk quantities of Jones and Bartlett's publications are available to corporations, professional associations, and other qualified organizations. For details and specific discount information, contact the special sales department at Jones and Bartlett via the above contact information or send an email to specialsales@jbpub.com.

The authors, editor, and publisher have made every effort to provide accurate information. However, they are not responsible for errors, omissions, or for any outcomes related to the use of the contents of this book and take no responsibility for the use of the products and procedures described. Treatments and side effects described in this book may not be applicable to all people; likewise, some people may require a dose or experience a side effect that is not described herein. Drugs and medical devices are discussed that may have limited availability controlled by the Food and Drug Administration (FDA) for use only in a research study or clinical trial. Research, clinical practice, and government regulations often change the accepted standard in this field. When consideration is being given to use of any drug in the clinical setting, the health care provider or reader is responsible for determining FDA status of the drug, reading the package insert, and reviewing prescribing information for the most up-to-date recommendations on dose, precautions, and contraindications, and determining the appropriate usage for the product. This is especially important in the case of drugs that are new or seldom used.

Production Credits
Executive Publisher: Christopher Davis
Editorial Assistant: Sara Cameron
Production Editor: Daniel Stone
V.P., Manufacturing and Inventory Control: Therese Connell
Manufacturing and Inventory Control Supervisor: Amy Bacus
Composition: International Typesetting and Composition
Cover Printing: Malloy, Inc.

Cover Credits
Cover Design: Carolyn Downer
Cover Printing: Malloy, Inc.
Cover Images: Top Image: © Sophie Louise Asselin/ShutterStock, Inc.; Bottom Right Image: Credit line: © T-Design/ShutterStock, Inc.; Bottom Right Image: © Luis Louro/ShutterStock, Inc.

Library of Congress Cataloging-in-Publication Data
Pass, Harvey I.
    100 questions & answers about mesothelioma/Harvey I. Pass, Amy Metula, Susan Vento.
    — 2nd ed.
        p. ; cm.
    Includes bibliographical references and index.
    ISBN-13: 978-0-7637-7123-2
    ISBN-10: 0-7637-7123-6
    1. Mesothelioma—Popular works. 2. Mesothelioma—Miscellanea. I. Metula, Amy.
    II. Vento, Susan. III. Title. IV. Title: One hundred questions & answers about mesothelioma.
    V. Title: One hundred questions and answers about mesothelioma.
    [DNLM: 1. Mesothelioma—Popular Works. QZ 340 P285z 2010]
    RC280.L8P375 2010
    616.99'424—dc22

                                                            2009018602
6048

Printed in the United States of America
13 12 01 10 09   10 9 8 7 6 5 4 3 2 1

Contents

Questions 1–7 address fundamental questions about mesothelioma, including the following:
- What is mesothelioma?
- What are the risk factors, or who gets mesothelioma?
- Can mesothelioma be prevented?

Questions 8–19 explain the methods used to detect and identify mesothelioma and the healthcare professionals involved in your diagnosis:
- What are the symptoms of mesothelioma, and how is it diagnosed?
- What tests are performed to help diagnose mesothelioma?
- Should I get a second opinion?

Questions 20–23 provide practical advice for dealing with the physical, emotional, and financial issues raised by a diagnosis of mesothelioma:
- What types of psychological support are available to me?
- What should my family know about mesothelioma in order to assist me?
- What about financial concerns and medical records?

Questions 24–32 discuss legal dimensions of the disease:
- I understand that mesothelioma and other asbestos-related diseases are controversial political issues. Why?
- How do I learn more about my rights?
- Do I need to have a will?

Contents

Orphan diseases like mesothelioma don't get the recognition they should, and when you have an orphan disease that is a political, economic, and health policy football, the situation becomes worse. Why? Because the patient gets lost in a confusing blame-game vortex, fortified by the lame arguments we have been hearing for the last 10 to 15 years:

- "It's an orphan disease that afflicts only 3000 per year; why put a lot of research dollars into it?"
- "It is caused by an environmental fiber that we have precautions against now, so once we get over this wave of cases we won't have to worry about it anymore."
- "Companies have gone bankrupt over this and can't afford to assume the health care burden of workers who contracted the disease through their employ."
- "It's a tort issue; the lawyers are making all the money through huge settlements, so we need to reform the system!"
- "People who have any injury from asbestos should be compensated fully, even if there isn't enough money for fair compensation of the mesothelioma victims."

The situation is also made worse by quotes like this from an influential academic: "I started my academic life treating mesothelioma and quickly learned that it was not very rewarding . . . Mesothelioma is a bear. We are better equipped going after . . . [other diseases] . . . where therapy makes a difference and we have expertise. We are not going very far chasing bears."

This is an intensely personal book on a personal issue—the lives of people with mesothelioma. I am just a surgeon whose second love is research. I saw only one mesothelioma patient in my training before I went to the National Institutes of Health (NIH). The NIH changed my life—there my career first intersected with ambition and then with true suffering. As a young, macho senior investigator who wanted to tinker with new therapeutic toys, using light to treat patients, I developed protocols for mesothelioma victims. During my time (HIP) at the NIH, I was on top of the world and strategically positioned to study mesothelioma: massive operations that only a few of us get to do, all the technical toys in the world, and all the mesothelioma patients to operate on, because very few surgeons really wanted to deal with the disease at that time.

All was good until I looked at the results of the early trials.

But really, the results of the trials are not the issue here. The issue is the people I met and touched, the ones in whom the disease recurred in seven months, the ones who looked at me in the clinic with their families, who came to me for help with their misery.

This book is to remind me of all those experiences of failure and of the days I spent beating my head against the wall trying to figure out why this killer is so smart. This book is to remind me of how many patients thanked me for my efforts when they knew they were dying, and of the ones who, after I told them that their disease had come back, asked me, "What do we do next, Dr. Pass?"

This book is a natural evolution for me, because the hotshot surgeon with all the answers had to be humbled before he felt worthy to give advice, and you certainly can't give advice until you have been sobered by experience.

I could not do a project like this unless I thought there was hope.

I truly believe that we are doing better for our mesothelioma patients now compared to when I was experimenting with photodynamic therapy. The reasons for these baby steps in improvement are many, including the training of young investigators who have recognized that mesothelioma is a fertile ground for novel therapies—young investigators who are a heck of a lot smarter than the dinosaurs of the previous generation, among whom I include myself. Collaborations are also occurring among the dinosaurs and the young investigators that were unheard of five years ago. Finally, there is a groundswell of activism for mesothelioma research on a national scale, which has spawned more (but not enough) NIH funding, independent grant awards from the Mesothelioma Applied Research Foundation, and blossoming pharmaceutical success stories, which, although modest, are truly significant improvements in therapy.

And then there are individuals like Bruce and Sue Vento. Sue can summarize her experience far more personally than any of us:

Although it's been many years since Bruce and I were first told that Bruce had mesothelioma, I can still hear those words as if they have just been uttered. It was a stunning moment. We knew it was cancer, but spelling and pronouncing it as well as understanding it were beyond us at that point. It's been an emotional journey. Along the way, I learned that family and friends and the love and support they provide are simply priceless. They are there when you need them most.

The health care professionals who dedicate their lives to working with cancer patients—especially mesothelioma patients—are a special breed of caring, highly skilled individuals. I will be forever grateful to them, and most especially to Dr. Dan Miller and his colleagues at the Mayo Clinic in Rochester. When they could no longer assist us, they advised us to secure hospice services, which we found from nurse Nancy Mullins and Father Gerald Foley and their colleagues at Healtheast Hospice Care in St. Paul.

Bruce and I were blessed in 2000 to be guided by three caring professionals: attorneys Mike Sieben and Tom Campbell and their staffs, who assisted us with asbestos litigation and with Bruce's will and living will, respectively, and Father John Malone, our priest and dear friend. On August 31, 2000, Father Malone married us with our family and friends present. The words from our vows, ". . . in sickness and in health, till death us do part" were especially meaningful and real for us. There was no way of knowing that Bruce would die forty days later. However, each and every one of those forty days was precious. I carry with me a picture of Bruce and the quote "Living life with a man you love is a life worth living." What a love; what a life.

Not everyone dies immediately from mesothelioma. While Bruce had only eight and one-half months to live following his diagnosis, since his death I have met people who have lived three, four, five, and six years since their own mesothelioma diagnoses, and they are looking and feeling great and are living full lives. This is a disease that can be corralled when diagnosed early and treated appropriately.

With a mesothelioma diagnosis, it doesn't take long to get one's priorities in order. I recall vividly the morning Bruce wanted oatmeal. After repeated failed attempts to make an edible bowl of oatmeal, I burst into tears. Bruce laughed. I realized then that together we could handle the challenges he faced. To this day, the many memories of his beaming smile and wonderful laugh warm my heart.

Finally, this is a senseless, cruel disease that doesn't have to exist, nor does it have to affect the lives of so many Americans. Joining with other mesothelioma survivors and their families, I will continue to work to reduce and eventually wipe out mesothelioma. Through concerted efforts, we can secure a federal ban on asbestos, funding for mesothelioma research, and increased resources to assist mesothelioma patients and their families.

I told you this is a very personal book.

It is written to try to guide; it is not written as a thesis. It is a distillation of "important things," as opposed to a collection of useless medical facts. It is meant to be personal for those who use it, and hopefully to cool that "rage-fear" reaction that you, the reader, are probably undergoing since you, or somebody you know, has been diagnosed with the disease. We want you to be better prepared to start on this unknown path, on which you must put your trust in strangers, who labor fiercely to destroy this orphan disease. Let this guide and the resources it contains show you that there are possibilities that offer hope and where to find them, and don't let the nihilism of others dissuade you from seeking the counsel of experienced mesothelioma clinicians. Make *informed* decisions—you owe it to yourself, and to the people who love you.

> *"Never doubt that a small group of thoughtful, committed citizens can change the world. Indeed, it's the only thing that ever has."*
>
> (Margaret Mead)

Harvey I. Pass, MD

PART ONE

The Basics

What is mesothelioma?

What are the risk factors, or
who gets mesothelioma?

Can mesothelioma be prevented?

More . . .

1. What is mesothelioma?

Pleura (PLOOR-a)

A thin layer of tissue covering the lungs and lining the interior wall of the chest cavity. It protects and cushions the lungs. This tissue secretes a small amount of fluid that acts as a lubricant, allowing the lungs to move smoothly in the chest cavity while breathing.

Peritoneum (PAIR-ih-toe-NEE-um)

The tissue that lines the abdominal wall and covers most of the organs in the abdomen which is composed of mesothelial cells and is the target organ for abdominal mesothelioma.

Pericardium

The heart sac that covers the heart.

Epithelial (ep-ih-THEE-lee-ul)

Refers to the cells that line the internal and external surfaces of the body and the term used to describe the appearance of the cells under the microsope for the most common type of mesothelioma.

Malignant mesothelioma is a rare form of cancer that is found in the lining of the chest and lung (the **pleura**), the abdomen (the **peritoneum**), or the saclike space around the heart (the **pericardium**). Although it is rare, mesothelioma is a very serious disease that is often at an advanced stage when the diagnosis is made.

In the United States an estimated 2000 to 3000 new cases of mesothelioma are diagnosed each year. Approximately three fourths of these cases start in the chest cavity and are called pleural mesotheliomas. Another 10% to 20% begin in the abdomen and are called peritoneal mesotheliomas. Lastly, those that start in the lining around the heart are called pericardial mesotheliomas, but these are extremely rare.

2. Are there different types of mesothelioma?

Mesothelioma is divided into three main types, based on what the cancer cells look like under the microscope. The most frequent type is **epithelioid**. About 50% to 70% of mesotheliomas are of this type. It usually has the best prognosis or outlook of the three. The second type is called the **sarcomatoid**, which makes up about 7% to 20% of mesotheliomas. It has a very unpredictable pattern or nature. The last type, called mixed or **biphasic**, is a combination of the first two types and makes up about 20% to 35% of mesotheliomas. Although there are different types of mesothelioma, the treatment options, at this time, are essentially the same for all types.

3. What is the pleura?

The pleura is a sheetlike lining formed by rectangular cells called mesothelial cells, and is usually not more than a few layers thick. There are two pleuras in the chest; the **parietal pleura** lines the inside of the chest wall like wallpaper, covering not only the inside of the ribs but also the diaphragm (the muscle in between the chest and abdominal cavities that moves with breathing) and pericardium. The normal parietal pleura is no more than 2 to 3 mm thick, where the normal **visceral pleura** is fused to the lung and is about 1 mm thick. The visceral pleura is a separate pleura that covers the lung and is much more difficult to remove without harming the lung. The pleura filters fluid back and forth from the chest to the circulation in the normal human, but it is expendable if it becomes diseased. If the pleura becomes diseased, it is not as effective in eliminating fluid from the chest, and fluid accumulation (pleural effusion) can occur.

4. What are the risk factors, or who gets mesothelioma?

In general, a risk factor is anything that can increase a person's chance of getting a particular disease. The biggest risk factor for developing mesothelioma is an exposure to asbestos. Most people with this disease have, at some point in their lives, worked on jobs where they breathed in asbestos fibers. The risk of developing mesothelioma is directly related to how much asbestos exposure a person has had and for how long. People who have a risk of occupational asbestos exposure include factory workers, ship builders, brake repair workers, construction workers, insulation manufacturers and installers, asbestos miners, and many others.

The Basics

Sarcomatoid

The least common variant of mesothelioma which has the appearance under the microscope of spindly cells which look like supportive or connective tissue.

Biphasic

A mesothelioma which has both epithelial and sarcomatoid elements. Also called a mixed mesothelioma.

Parietal pleura

The lining on the inside of the chest wall which is composed of mesothelial cells and is the target organ for asbestos induced mesothelioma.

Visceral pleura

The mesothelial living on the surface of the lung which can also be a target organ for mesothelioma.

Family members of people exposed to asbestos at work are also at an increased risk for mesothelioma. This is because these asbestos fibers are carried home on the clothes, shoes, skin, and hair of these workers and can be inhaled by others.

Simian virus 40, or SV40, is a virus that has been associated with the development of malignant mesothelioma. This virus is found in rhesus monkeys and is now widespread among humans. The way this virus was transferred from monkeys to humans is uncertain, but it is postulated that some of the transfer occurred from 1954 to 1963 through SV40-contaminated polio vaccines administered worldwide. Those people who received the injectable form of the polio vaccine are believed to be those at greatest risk. This vaccine doesn't fully explain the transfer of this virus, because many humans who could not have received the contaminated vaccines are now infected with the SV40 virus. One theory that has been proposed is that the SV40 virus continues to be transferred from monkeys to humans or that humans can pass the virus from person to person. The latter theory has been supported by data showing that SV40 can be excreted in human feces, breast milk, and semen. It is unlikely that this virus acts alone in the development of mesothelioma as most cancers have multiple risk factors associated with their development, and most mesotheliomas occur in asbestos exposed individuals. Instead, it is more likely that asbestos and SV40 may act together to develop into mesothelioma.

Although rare, cases of mesothelioma have been found following radiation exposure to the chest and abdomen. These individuals were usually treated in the past with radiation therapy for a malignancy of the lymph glands known as lymphoma.

Lastly, there is an indication that a person's own genes can play an important role in determining who is susceptible, or vulnerable, to these mineral fibers and will then develop mesothelioma. It is hoped that doctors will be able to find the specific susceptibility gene in the future and that this may lead to the development of new prevention and treatment strategies to better control this disease.

Sue adds . . .

Having taught for seven years, and in my current role working with and for public school teachers and educational support professionals in Minnesota, I was stunned to learn of the number of individuals who were exposed to asbestos in school settings. Equally stunning is the number of people who were unknowingly exposed while serving in the military as well as while doing home remodeling and repair projects.

5. What causes mesothelioma?

Exposure to asbestos is the link to the development of mesothelioma. People who end up with this disease usually have had some type of previous exposure to asbestos. How this works is not fully understood. It is thought that asbestos fibers are inhaled and first travel through the upper air passages, which include the throat, the trachea (windpipe), and the large bronchi (large breathing tubes of the lungs). These airways are lined with mucus, and therefore most of the fibers are cleared from these upper airways by sticking to this mucus and being coughed up or swallowed. When the fibers continue to travel and reach the small airways (the alveoli), the body's immune system is able to surround, engulf, and remove the smaller fibers by a process known as phagocytosis. The large, long, thin fibers cannot be cleared as easily and may eventually reach the pleura (the lining of the lung and the chest wall), where they may irritate and injure the cells and lead to the development of calcium containing plate-like structures on the pleural lining (pleural plaques), fibrosis (scar tissue formation), or mesothelioma. These same asbestos fibers can also damage cells in the lung itself, which can lead to asbestosis (scar tissue in the lung) and/or lung cancer. Patients with these pleural plaques seem to be at highest risk for developing mesothelioma.

6. Can mesothelioma be prevented?

The best way to prevent mesothelioma is to decrease one's exposure to asbestos in the workplace, at home, and in the environment. The federal government is responsible for developing regulations that deal with asbestos exposure in the workplace. The agency that issues these regulations is known as the Occupational Safety and Health Administration (OSHA). Employers are required to follow these regulations, and therefore workers who are concerned about asbestos exposure should be discussing these concerns with their employers or union. Also, employees should be using all protective equipment provided to them by their employers and following recommended safety procedures and practices while at work.

If you are exposed to asbestos in the workplace, you should be aware of the potential of bringing the fibers home on your clothes, skin, and hair. It is best to change your clothes and shower at work if at all possible. If not, then it is important to do this immediately upon arriving home, which will limit the amount of exposure to others. Remove your clothes and put them in the washing machine as soon as possible.

Don't forget! Asbestos is associated with lung cancer too! Many studies have shown that the combination of smoking and exposure to asbestos is particularly hazardous. The risk of lung cancer is greatly increased in asbestos-exposed individuals who smoke. However, smoking in the absence of asbestos exposure has not been associated with the development of mesothelioma. Nevertheless, did you know that certain cigarette filters were constructed from asbestos fibers? Fortunately, this brand, Kents, is no longer on the market.

Because of the combined effect of smoking and asbestos exposure, it is important for anyone who has ever been exposed to asbestos, or who suspects that he or she may have been exposed to the fibers, to quit smoking, or not to start. People who have been exposed to asbestos should also get regular physical exams and should seek prompt medical treatment for any respiratory illnesses.

7. What is asbestos?

Asbestos is a naturally occurring group of minerals that have been mined and used in different industries since the late 1800s. It is an extremely poor conductor of heat and does not conduct electricity, and therefore it has been widely used as an insulator. The flexible asbestos fibers are woven after being separated into thin threads. The fibers tend to break easily, and the dust that is formed from them breaking can float in the air and stick to clothes. The fibers can also be inhaled or swallowed and can result in serious health problems, including asbestosis, lung cancer, and mesothelioma.

There are six types of asbestos: amosite, crocidolite, anthophyllite, actinolite, tremolite, and chrysotile. The first five types are called amphibole asbestos, and they all have needlelike fibers. Chrysotile has a different texture, composition, and behavior than amphibole asbestos. Although some findings suggest that amphibole asbestos is more cancer causing than chrysotile, the topic remains controversial.

Recently, other types of mined minerals have been found to be associated with asbestos, including vermiculite and taconite. Vermiculite has been used in insulation, and recently there has been great concern that it can be associated with mesothelioma. Vermiculite is also mixed into soil to lighten it and make it more porous, for gardening. Vermiculite mining was performed in Libby, Montana, and the number of mesothelioma cases reported in that community has increased significantly. Moreover, many homes across the nation have used vermiculite for insulation.

PART TWO

Diagnosis

What are the symptoms of mesothelioma,
and how is it diagnosed?

What tests are performed to help
diagnose mesothelioma?

Should I get a second opinion?

More . . .

8. What are the symptoms of mesothelioma?

Latency period

The time between the actual exposure to a carcinogen like asbestos and the development of cancer, i.e. mesothelioma.

Mesothelioma has a very long **latency period** (the time from the initial asbestos exposure to the development of cancer), making it doubly treacherous. This latency period can be anywhere from 25 to 40 years. The length of time it takes patients to report symptoms varies but can range from two weeks to two years, with the average being about two months. As many as 25% of patients with the disease can have symptoms for six months or more before seeking medical attention. Due to its slow onset, the disease tends to affect people between 50 and 70 years of age. It affects men three to five times more often than women and is less common in African Americans than in Caucasians. The right side of the chest is affected more than the left. The right lung is bigger than the left lung, or the right lung is of greater size and volume than the left lung.

Chest pain

Discomfort in the chest that can be a feeling of "heaviness" to a constant boring pain requiring narcotics.

Dyspnea

Difficult, painful breathing or shortness of breath. One of the early symptoms of mesothelioma in the pleura due to the accumulation of fluid in the chest.

Pleural effusion

An abnormal collection of fluid between the thin layers of tissue (pleura) lining the lung and the wall of the chest cavity.

The most common features associated with the development of symptoms include the presence of fluid, thickening of the pleura, and specific nodules or tumors that may develop in the chest or abdomen. Over half of the patients have **chest pain,** usually located low in the chest and toward the back and side. The pain has usually increased over time and can be severe enough to require narcotic pain medication. Severe, uncontrolled pain may be a sign of tumor invasion into the chest wall. The chest wall refers to the structures outside the lungs that move as a part of breathing, including the rib cage and diaphragm. **Dyspnea** (difficulty breathing) is another symptom commonly seen with this disease. This shortness of breath is usually due to fluid that has accumulated in the pleural space (the space between the chest wall and the lung) from the cancer. This fluid accumulation is called a **pleural effusion.** In 95% of the cases, patients with pleural mesothelioma will have a pleural effusion at some time during the course of the disease. Cough, fever, fatigue, and weight loss will occur in about 30% of cases, and a small minority will have hoarseness or will cough up blood **(hemoptysis)**. In only about 5% will the disease have spread out of the initial area of cancer **(metastasis),** usually traveling from the pleura spreading to the lungs, which can cause these last symptoms to occur.

In abdominal or peritoneal mesothelioma, patients most frequently have increased abdominal swelling from fluid that has accumulated in the abdomen **(ascites)**. They may also have pain and weight loss. Pain in the abdomen is usually due to an increase in the amount of solid tumor they have, and not because of fluid. Weight loss can be due to a decreased appetite because of the disease.

Sue adds . . .

Until just two weeks before Bruce's diagnosis, he had not shown any symptoms of serious illness. He began the new millennium with the intention of completing his 12th term in Congress, running for his 13th, and, most importantly, welcoming his fifth grandchild, who was born in May. His first symptoms surfaced while on a trip in mid–January and were a severe shortness of breath and discomfort in his back. Bruce had always been quite active, bicycling, swimming, or working out on the Nautilus daily.

9. How is mesothelioma diagnosed?

If you experience shortness of breath, pain in the chest or abdomen, swelling in the abdomen, or any other unusual symptom, see your doctor! The doctor will take a history from you and perform a physical exam. In listening to your chest, the doctor may not hear

Hemoptysis
Coughing up blood.

Metastasis (meh-TAS-ta-sis)
The spread of cancer from one part of the body to another. A tumor formed by cells that have spread is called a "metastatic tumor" or a "metastasis." The metastatic tumor contains cells that are like those in the original (primary) tumor. The plural form of metastasis is metastases (meh-TAS-ta-seez).

Ascites (ah-SYE-teez)
Abnormal build-up of fluid in the abdomen that may cause swelling. In late-stage cancer, tumor cells may be found in the fluid in the abdomen. Ascites is a common manifestation of peritoneal mesothelioma and can occur as a manifestation of recurrent mesothelioma after surgery for the disease in the chest.

breath sounds clearly on one side or may hear scratchy sounds in the chest (rub). Or the doctor may notice that your abdomen is swollen. After the examination, the doctor will link the symptoms you reported to the findings on the physical exam. The doctor will want to know whether you have had other symptoms, like fever, chills, pain, or unusual lumps on the torso. The doctor will also want to know whether your appetite is good and whether you have lost any weight. He or she may ask about asbestos exposure and cigarette use.

After performing the physical exam and taking a history that concentrates on whether you have developed shortness of breath or pain, the doctor will order a chest x-ray. Based on what is found, the doctor will determine what other tests you will need. The doctor may also order blood work. When a tumor or fluid is found, the doctor will need to perform a procedure that will obtain cells for the physicians to study to determine whether this is a cancer or not. This can be done by performing a biopsy of the mass or by tapping fluid (inserting a needle and drawing out fluid) from the chest or belly cavity and then analyzing the cells that come with the fluid. The analysis of cells from fluid is called **cytology**. Although an x-ray or scan may provide useful information about the size, shape, and location of a tumor or fluid and may alert your doctor to the possibility of a cancer, an actual diagnosis of mesothelioma cannot be made without a biopsy, or undeniable evidence of cells in the fluid that have the characteristics of a mesothelioma.

Cytology

The study of cells using a microscope.

10. Are blood tests useful to diagnose mesothelioma?

There are no specific blood tests that can tell your doctor you have mesothelioma. Certain blood cell values may be abnormal when a patient has mesothelioma, but these are nonspecific (that is, they do not definitively tell the doctor that it is mesothelioma or another type of cancer or a benign condition). The **white blood cell** count (cells that fight infection) may be elevated and/or the **platelet** count (cells that help the clotting system) may be elevated above normal values.

The liquid part of blood (serum) is partially comprised of dissolved proteins. Currently, there are no specific proteins in the serum that can tell your doctor you have asbestosis or mesothelioma. Proteins that are specific to a certain disease are called biomarkers. There is great interest in the discovery of these **biomarkers**, which may represent unique proteins from the tumor that appear early in the disease and increase as the disease progresses. Ask your physician whether any of these markers are under study or whether any have been approved by the FDA for the study of mesothelioma. These markers include soluble mesothelin related protein (SMRP) and osteopontin.

11. What tests are performed to help diagnose mesothelioma?

As we mentioned previously, the first test that is usually performed after the history and physical exam is an x-ray of the chest. These x-rays can show areas of fluid accumulation, scarring of the lungs, masses in the chest, and other types of abnormal findings, but they are not as sensitive as other tests available today.

The results of the chest x-ray will usually prompt the doctor to order a CAT or CT scan (computerized axial tomography scan) of the chest and abdomen. These scans provide a three-dimensional view of the area of

Diagnosis

White blood cell (WBC)

Refers to a blood cell that does not contain hemoglobin. White blood cells include lymphocytes, neutrophils, eosinophils, macrophages, and mast cells. These cells are made by bone marrow and help the body fight infection and other diseases.

Platelet (PLAYT-let)

A type of blood cell that helps prevent bleeding by causing blood clots to form. Also called a thrombocyte.

Biomarker

A substance sometimes found in the blood, other body fluids, or tissues. A high level of biomarker may mean that a certain type of cancer is in the body. Examples of biomarkers include CA 125 (ovarian cancer), CA 15-3 (breast cancer), CEA (ovarian, lung, breast, pancreas, and gastrointestinal tract cancers), and PSA (prostate cancer). Also called tumor marker.

CAT scan

A series of detailed pictures of areas inside the body, taken from different angles; the pictures are created by a computer linked to an x-ray machine. Also called computerized axial tomography, computed tomography (CT scan), or computerized tomography.

Magnetic resonance imaging (mag-NET-ik REZ-o-nans IM-a-jing) (MRI)

A procedure in which radio waves and a powerful magnet linked to a computer are used to create detailed pictures of areas inside the body. These pictures can show the difference between normal and diseased tissue. MRI makes better images of organs and soft tissue than other scanning techniques, such as CT or x-ray. MRI is especially useful for imaging the brain, spine, the soft tissue of joints, and the inside of bones. Also called nuclear magnetic resonance imaging.

the body that the physician is interested in. **CT scans** have a better ability to show how much solid mass is present and how much fluid contributes to the picture. They also give a much better anatomic picture so your doctor can see how any masses relate to the lung, heart, diaphragm (the muscle that helps you breathe), and blood vessels in the chest or abdomen. CT scans do not tell the doctor what type of tumor it is or whether the disease has invaded other structures, but they do give a very good idea of whether your disease can be classified as early with minimal disease (Stage I), later with moderate amount of disease (Stage II), or advanced with a large amount of disease (Stages III and IV). (We will discuss the concept of staging in more detail later on.) In mesothelioma, a CT scan is not very good for showing whether your lymph nodes (the round structures in certain positions in the chest and abdomen that drain the lung and intestines and act as filters and sites for immune responses) are involved. The reason it does not show this well is that the pleura can be thickened in areas where the lymph nodes are, and this lumpy, bumpy thickening can be confused with lymph nodes or can hide lymph nodes.

The doctor may also request an MRI (**magnetic resonance image**). An MRI uses radio waves and strong magnets along with a computer to form detailed images of the body. The MRI can occasionally give the doctor information about whether the diaphragm or chest wall have become involved and if the tumor has invaded through it. Not all mesothelioma specialists use MRIs in their workup.

A **PET scan** (positron emission tomography scan) is a relatively new type of scan that shows how the body takes up and uses glucose (sugar). Tumors, cancer cells, and areas that are inflamed or infected use glucose at a higher rate than normal tissues do. Since a radioactive tracer is attached to the glucose injected into your body, the areas which use glucose at a higher rate (i.e. tumors) will hold onto the radioactive tracer longer than normal cells. Areas on PET scans that "light up" as bright spots are abnormal. It is important to know, however, that abnormal areas on PET scans are not necessarily cancerous; they can also be the result of inflammation. The PET scan can also give the doctor information as to whether the cancer has spread outside the original area to other parts of the body, and it may pick up areas of spread that are completely unexpected. There have not been enough large studies that prove the usefulness of this scan in mesothelioma, and therefore it has not been approved by most insurance companies as a standard test for mesothelioma, as it has been for lung cancer. However, there are mechanisms that can help pay for PET scans that doctors who do them (nuclear medicine physicians) can help you with. Ask them about these programs.

Your doctor will also order a biopsy when a tumor or fluid is suspected to be cancerous.

12. How are biopsies performed, and which biopsy is best for me?

A patient with a large, unexplained fluid accumulation in the chest or abdomen and who has a small or moderate amount of thickening of the pleura should have a biopsy performed, using semi-invasive techniques (techniques that require only local anesthesia and that do not involve cutting into the chest or abdomen). For example, the biopsy might involve an initial **thoracentesis** (drainage of fluid in the chest) or **paracentesis** (drainage

PET scan

Positron emission tomography scan. A procedure in which a small amount of radioactive glucose (sugar) is injected into a vein, and a scanner is used to make detailed, computerized pictures of areas inside the body where the glucose is used. Because cancer cells often use more glucose than normal cells, the pictures can be used to find cancer cells in the body.

Thoracentesis (thor-a-sen-TEE-sis)

Removal of fluid from the pleural cavity through a needle inserted between the ribs.

Paracentesis

Insertion of a thin needle or tube into the abdomen to remove fluid from the peritoneal cavity. Commonly used to make the diagnosis of peritoneal mesothelioma in patients with ascites or to diagnose recurrence of the disease in the belly.

of fluid in the abdomen) and a pleural **biopsy**. These are relatively safe procedures that can be performed by a pulmonologist (lung physician), a radiologist, or a surgeon. A **local anesthetic** (a numbing medicine such as lidocaine) is given to temporarily reduce the feeling in the area before the needle is inserted.

A pleural biopsy with a special needle may help in getting a diagnosis of mesothelioma, and it is generally performed by a pulmonologist. Since mesothelioma is usually diffuse (widely scattered) in the chest, a random sample of the pleura may give tissue with mesothelioma cells in it.

A thoracentesis can be performed after the pleural biopsy is completed. The doctor inserts a needle into the pocket of fluid in the chest or abdomen to draw off some of the fluid. Many times, the needle is simply used to insert a flexible catheter (a tube the size of thin spaghetti) which is then used to draw off the fluid. After the fluid is drawn out through this catheter, the catheter is removed.

The fluid and the tissue from the pleural biopsy will be sent to a pathologist and/or cytologist who will look under the microscope at the cells and determine whether mesothelioma is present. In the past, a diagnosis of mesothelioma from fluid alone was possible only a third of the time because of the difficulty of distinguishing between reactive or noncancerous cells and tumor cells. By staining the fluid with a special substance, pathologists can now make a diagnosis more easily. Your doctor will refer to these stains as "immunos," short for immunohistochemistry. You should make sure that any material used in the biopsy has been studied using these immuno stains. A chest x-ray is always performed after these procedures to make sure there were no complications from the biopsies, such as an accumulation of air in the chest (pneumothorax). The chest x-ray is also very important to see whether the majority of the fluid has been removed and if the lung is now able to expand with air and fill the chest cavity, as it normally should.

More-invasive testing may be needed if the initial results of the semi-invasive tests do not provide adequate information or if the CT scan indicates that it would be difficult to do the semi-invasive tests. The latter situation would occur if the fluid is not free flowing but is hidden in pockets that are difficult to reach. In such cases, it is better to inspect the chest directly to find out where to do the biopsy. A **thoracoscopy** (the use of a lighted scope, with or without a camera, to look into the chest) is performed in patients who are at risk for mesothelioma and who develop a large fluid accumulation, with or without associated solid tumor masses in the chest. In patients who are at risk for mesothelioma but whose thoracentesis does not reveal cancer cells, or who experience a recurrence of fluid after the initial thoracentesis is performed, a thoracoscopy should probably be performed. This procedure involves using a special lighted instrument called a thoracoscope to look inside the chest cavity. The scope is placed into the chest between two ribs after a small (1-inch) cut is made through the chest wall. If the doctor finds any tissue that looks abnormal, he or she will cut out a piece, or biopsy a piece, of it to have it looked at under the microscope. This tissue will then be examined for cancer cells.

A thoracoscopy can provide information crucial for deciding how to treat the patient. It gives great insight

Thoracoscopy

The use of a thin, lighted tube (called an endoscope) to examine the inside of the chest.

Diagnosis

into the amount of disease that is present as well as where the disease is present—for example, on the parietal pleura alone or on both the parietal pleura and the visceral pleura, on the diaphragm, or on the pericardium. The status of the lung can also be assessed with a thoracoscopy. For example, it will show whether the lung does not expand because it has a concretelike layer of tumor on it which restricts the lung from filling with air with each breath. A laparoscopy is similar to a thoracoscopy but involves looking into the abdomen.

Peritoneoscopy

The use of a thin lighted tube (called a laparoscope to examine the abdomen).

Lastly, if the radiologic tests indicate that there is more solid tumor than fluid, or if there is no longer a space where fluid can accumulate because of previous attempts to control the fluid, an "open" biopsy may be indicated. The incision does not have to be large if the pleura is thickened, but the procedure should be performed by a thoracic surgeon who understands the principles of mesothelioma treatment. This surgeon will usually suggest a 3- or 4-inch incision on the side of the chest, overlying an area of pleura that is thickened. The surgeon may or may not remove a small piece of rib at this site to allow a direct view of the thickened pleura. Many times, a good-sized piece of pleura (1 to 1 1/2 inches in diameter) can be removed at this site. Getting a quick freeze of the tissue in the operating room, with the pathologist looking at the biopsy, will ensure that there's enough tissue to perform all the required testing and to make a diagnosis. Surgeons performing these biopsies should pick the right place for the biopsy, and the cut (incision) for this biopsy should be in line with the longer incision that would be used later if the patient is a surgical candidate. That way, this shorter incision can be removed.

Although this operation is performed under general anesthesia (putting the patient to sleep), many times a chest tube to drain the air out of the chest is not needed because the surgeon never enters the chest cavity itself. The patient may need some pain medicine for about a week after the procedure if he or she was not having pain before the biopsy.

Finally, mesothelioma can "set up shop" and grow tumors at biopsy sites. Radiation therapy is sometimes used after a thoracoscopy or open biopsy to prevent the disease from growing at those sites. If the biopsy results indicate mesothelioma, discuss this option with your physician.

13. How will I learn about my biopsy results, and how can I be sure the diagnosis is mesothelioma?

After a biopsy is completed, the tissue or fluid is sent to a specialized doctor called a **pathologist**. Pathologists' field of study is the origin and cause of disease. They look at the cells from biopsies under the microscope and are responsible for deciding whether cancer cells are present. The pathologist who studies your biopsy will generate a report about what he or she has found and send it to your doctor. This usually takes about five days to complete. You should make an appointment for a follow-up office visit with your doctor after this time period. He or she will then go over the pathologist's results with you. It is important to bring someone along with you to this appointment if possible. This person can help you remember all the information that is given to you by your doctor, which can sometimes be overwhelming. He or she can also be a support to you during this stressful period.

Pathologist (pa-THOL-o-jist)

A doctor who identifies diseases by studying cells and tissues under a microscope.

You need to make sure that the diagnosis in your case is correct, and you have every right to ask certain specific questions about the biopsy. Since mesothelioma is not a common disease, your primary doctor should make sure that all the appropriate testing has been performed on the specimen, including special stains (those immunos we talked about before), in order to distinguish mesothelioma from other cancers like adenocarcinoma of the lung. If there is any question, a common practice is to send the slides of the biopsy to specialists in mesothelioma, who can consult (*re-read the slides to confirm the report*) and render an opinion on the case. *You should ask your doctor to have the slides read in consultation by pathologists who are specific experts in mesothelioma.*

14. I have been given a diagnosis of mesothelioma. Since this is a rare disease, how do I know that my physicians have enough experience with the disease to treat me?

It is important that you get the best information available regarding your particular condition in order to decrease confusion, establish confidence in the treatment team, and have every opportunity to fight the disease and live as long as possible. In the majority of cases, your physician will inform you whether the institution he or she is associated with has a special interest in the disease and treats more than 50 cases of mesothelioma per year. If those resources are not at your physician's disposal, he or she should recommend a second opinion at a **cancer center**, which is a specialized institution to which he can refer you for mesothelioma. You should not lose your primary physician or the physician who made this initial diagnosis as your advocates. He or she will play a crucial

Cancer center

A hospital that specializes only in the care of patients with cancer. An NCI designated cancer center is specifically recognized and partially funded by the National Cancer Institute.

role in coordinating your care with the cancer center by making the initial contact (**referral**), and often by coordinating the testing to be done close to your home, so that when you visit the cancer center much of the workup will already have been performed.

15. Should I get a second opinion?

It is always a good idea to get a second opinion so that you know about every option available to you. The first physician you see about the disease may not be an expert in the field of mesothelioma. Having a second opinion allows you to seek out those with knowledge of the disease and its treatment. Also, different cancer centers may have different treatment options available. When you seek consultation with other physicians, the mesothelioma expert should inform you and your family of what is available to you. Remember, you have a right to choose where you go for treatment and what physician will ultimately be responsible for your care. It is important that you feel comfortable with the health care team, as they will be assisting you along the way with many important decisions. If your primary doctor, or the oncologist that you have been referred to, is not a mesothelioma specialist, ask about a second opinion at a mesothelioma center. Your doctors should be open to such a suggestion; if they are not, seek other sources that can help you find a mesothelioma expert.

16. How do I go about getting a second opinion?

If you decide that you want to get a second opinion, you must first check with your insurance company to see if your plan includes coverage for second opinions and the physician you plan to see. You may have to ask the insurance company for a referral to see another

Referral

A primary physician seeks expert consultation in cases by referring the patient to a specialist who may or may not be associated with a cancer center.

doctor if you have an HMO or a similar managed care organization. If you are a member of such a health care delivery system, your choices may be limited. These companies will provide you with a list of physicians who are within their network and ask you to choose from this list. You may have to request special permission to see a specialist out of the network if the physician you want to see is not one of those listed.

Next, make an appointment to see the physician you choose as soon as possible. You will need to have your insurance information and social security number available, as the specialist's office will ask for this when making the appointment. The specialist's office will also request that you bring all medical information, test results, biopsy slides, and x-ray/CT films with you to the appointment. These can all be signed out from your primary care doctor's office as well as from the medical records department, x-ray/CT film room, and pathology department of the hospital in which you received your care. If you need assistance with this, ask the office staff to help you. It is important that if you are traveling a long distance to see the specialist, you have as complete a copy of the materials as possible. Also make sure you ask about bringing not only reports but also the actual films or compact discs (CDs) that have all your films on them, as well as the glass slides from the biopsy, so the specialists' pathology department can make its own reading.

17. Who treats mesothelioma?

Oncology is a branch of medicine that deals with cancer, and an oncologist is a specialized doctor who treats people with these cancers. Depending on your particular treatment plan and which cancer center you are referred to, you may be seen first by a **medical oncologist**

Medical oncologist

A specially certified physician who treats cancer and delivers chemotherapy.

(a specially certified physician who treats cancer and delivers chemotherapy), a **thoracic surgical oncologist** (a general thoracic surgeon whose practice is almost exclusively the treatment of cancers in the chest and who does not perform heart surgery), or a **radiation oncologist** (a physician who delivers radiation). Mesothelioma is a very rare disease and therefore should be managed by doctors who have experience in treating it. The ideal situation is to be referred to a cancer center that deals with the disease in a multimodal way. That is, one that has a team of physicians from medicine, surgery, and radiation; nurses; and pain specialists who meet and discuss every patient in an individualized fashion. This group of specialists is called the multidisciplinary team. The key words here are "experience" and "protocols." You should insist on seeing individuals experienced in treating mesothelioma and who offer clinical trials (protocols) studying new ways to treat the disease.

18. How do I find the best doctors to treat my mesothelioma?

In order to find the best doctors to treat your disease, it is important to do some research, unless your physician is very well versed in the mesothelioma treatment landscape. The best place to start is with a computer that has access to the Internet. If you don't have a computer at home, you can go to any public library, where someone can assist you. It is important to find out where the mesothelioma centers are located and how close these centers are to you. The resources section after Question 100 lists web sites of interest. These centers have doctors who specialize in this disease. Your family doctor or internist may be able to help you locate someone as well. It is mandatory to do "due diligence" on any doctor you may decide to see, to find

Thoracic surgical oncologist

A general thoracic surgeon whose practice is almost exclusively the treatment of cancers in the chest and who does not perform heart surgery.

Radiation oncologist

A physician who delivers radiation.

Diagnosis

out about his or her experience and credentials. It is also a good idea to educate yourself about the disease and its treatment, so keep reading!

19. What can I do to make my doctor visits as productive as possible?

It is important that you and your doctor communicate clearly and understand each other well. Before you visit a center or a specific doctor, see whether either has a website that you can visit. You may be pleasantly surprised that a lot of your questions about the place or physician you are visiting are dealt with on this website. Nevertheless, how comfortable you are with your doctor will determine what questions you are able to ask and how successful your visit will be. If you don't understand something that your doctor tells you, let him or her know this! You should be able to receive the information in a form that is understandable to you. Ask the doctor to speak in simple terms if you find the language too complex. If you have concerns about anything that is said, speak up and discuss these issues. Take the time to repeat back to the doctor what you heard so that he or she knows what information to reinforce and what to correct. Talk with your doctor about what your knowledge is of the disease and its treatment and any concerns and/or fears you may have. Try to have discussions in a quiet, private place so that you don't become distracted. It is always a good idea to write out a list of questions that you would like to ask before coming to an appointment. If you don't receive an answer to a question, you may have to ask it more than once until you get an answer. If you are having trouble asking a specific question, you may want to ask to speak to the nurse or social worker. They are wonderful resources for you and are very approachable. Also, ask your health care team for any education materials, web sites, or other sources of information that may help you with your disease and its treatment. Get business cards from everybody so you know how to reach them!

Sue adds . . . .

Having a notebook plus a replacement notebook or two with you each time you meet with health care professionals will be a valuable tool for you in keeping track of all the information, terminology, medications, and instructions. Your spouse or friend can take thorough notes about the diagnosis, recommendations regarding care, medication, future appointments, and so forth. Don't hesitate to ask health care professionals to repeat and/or define medical terminology and specific procedures and instructions. Listing important phone numbers inside the front cover or on the first few pages of the notebook is also recommended— include the doctor's receptionist, scheduler, and after-hour numbers as well as numbers for the pharmacist and other health care professionals.

PART THREE

Coping

What types of psychological support
are available to me?

What should my family know about
mesothelioma in order to assist me?

What about financial concerns
and medical records?

More . . .

20. What types of psychosocial support are available to me?

A "health care team" is made up of many individuals who can provide support to you. These include doctors, nurses, social workers, counselors, and any other professionals you may see during your illness. They are very willing to help you deal with the diagnosis in any way possible. Don't hesitate to call on them when you need to.

Support groups are one way of communicating with others who have had similar experiences, and they are an excellent source of information for you. Unfortunately, because mesothelioma is such a rare disease, there has been a lack of specific support groups for these patients. Instead, they have had to rely on support groups that deal with other types of cancers. However, a few foundations, such as the Mesothelioma Applied Research Foundation (www.curemeso.org), specifically deal with the disease and can offer advice or point you in the right direction. Ask for a list of any groups in your area. Also, your doctor can give you the names and phone numbers of some patients with mesothelioma that he or she has treated. Many patients are willing and eager to share their experiences with others and may provide excellent support to you. They are able to provide a patient's point of view and share personal experiences they have had. This enables you to have a better understanding of what the process may be like and what you can expect before treatment even starts.

Sue adds . . .

Because of the increased awareness of mesothelioma and other diseases caused by asbestos, patient/family support groups are forming in various parts of the country. Don't hesitate to check the phone book or the Internet or to ask your physician or attorney or others to see if such an organization is available to you. Many of the victims and family members who have faced this diagnosis will be most happy to talk with you and will welcome your call with lots of helpful insights and endless support.

21. What should my family know about mesothelioma in order to assist me?

Telling family members about a diagnosis of mesothelioma is a difficult thing to do. They may experience a lot of the same emotions that you do, including fear, worry, concern, anger, and sadness. These emotions need to be expressed, even when they are strong. The best recommendation is to communicate openly and honestly with one another. This enables you and your family to cope better with the cancer diagnosis. The entire adult family should discuss all aspects of the disease before you start treatment. This includes the type of mesothelioma, the prognosis, treatment options, goals of treatment, and side effects expected. If a family member has specific questions that cannot be answered within the group or requires more in-depth information, he or she should feel free to call the doctor to discuss these issues, and should feel that the doctor is happy to inform him or her so that everybody will be on the same wavelength!

Sue adds . . .

A telephone tree/phone chain (see Appendix B) is very helpful in keeping family and friends informed. It will allow you to make two to four calls, or as many calls as necessary to get the update message started; those contacts then can contact others on the tree. Such updates can include suggestions as to whether or not it's advisable to call and/or visit, and if so, when. Whether the visits are to the hospital or home, it's important for loved ones to know that recovery from the surgery and aftereffects of chemotherapy and radiation can be quite exhausting. Visits may need to be rescheduled and should be brief and quiet. For those loved ones who want to help in other ways, keep a list of "to do's" and share them with those who offer. Tackling routine tasks—cleaning, yard work, auto upkeep, laundry, and so on—as well as day-to-day errands will be an energy and time saver for the care provider and is a wonderful gift.

22. What insurance and financial concerns do I need to address following a mesothelioma diagnosis?

When you are faced with a medical diagnosis of cancer, there are many issues that come to the forefront. One important consideration is your insurance coverage. Having health care insurance does decrease the financial burden that is placed upon you; however, even with good insurance, health care costs can be high. It is important to find out what your particular insurance plan covers and what you will be held responsible for paying. All health plans are not created equal in this regard, and the amount you may have to pay can vary widely. Don't assume that something will be paid for without first thoroughly investigating the situation. It is necessary to understand your health care policy before starting any treatment plan so that there are no surprises.

23. What should I know about medical records, and how do I manage them?

It is a good idea to keep a personal copy of all your medical records in a file so that you can access them when needed. It becomes difficult to remember every-thing that has happened to you over the course of your illness, and having these records is a good way to keep things organized. You can obtain a copy of your records by contacting the medical records department of the hospital and/or clinic where you have received or are currently receiving treatment. Also, you can request medical records from your doctor's office. To obtain your records, you may have to sign a written request form and pay a fee for the service. You will want to get copies of all the tests you have had, includ-ing lab and x-ray/CT scan reports, as well as any treat-ment records. This will provide you with a full health history of all your experiences right at your fingertips. If you have to see another doctor or specialist at some time in the future, you can bring a copy of your records with you so the doctor has a full understanding of your medical history. You should add to your files a list of the medications you are on and any side effects that may have occurred with them. Maintaining a sense of direction during this stressful time is imperative, and organization can help maintain that sense of direction. Keeping your resources, reports, contacts, and treat-ment history will help you locate information when-ever necessary.

Sue adds . . .

Having a central file—a box, file folder, or drawer—for all insurance and medical records will be a time-saver. When in doubt about any of the records, do not hesitate to call the care provider or insurer. Typically, toll-free num-bers are included on all statements and communications.

PART FOUR

The Politics of Mesothelioma

I understand that mesothelioma and other asbestos-related diseases are controversial political issues. Why?

How do I learn more about my legal rights?

Do I need to have a will?

More . . .

24. I understand that mesothelioma and other asbestos-related diseases are controversial political issues. Why?

Since the early 1900s, the truth about asbestos and the diseases it causes has been known and hidden from the American public. The U.S. and Canada are the only remaining Western countries that have not yet made significant efforts to halt the use and trade of asbestos. Too many believe that asbestos was banned a long time ago and/or that lengthy, intense exposure is needed to cause illness. Both of those beliefs are absolutely false.

Since the beginning of the millennium, the news media, authors, and government agencies and officials have paid increasing attention to asbestos and the diseases it causes throughout the country due to legislative proposals in Congress and due to asbestos related incidents in communities throughout the country. There have been political debates regarding the litigation against asbestos manufacturers and the financial impact it has on those companies and their insurers. Those debates have subsided a bit since 2006, when legislation to create a federal trust did not pass. Since then there have been increased efforts to pass legislation to ban the use and distribution of asbestos in the U.S., to increase public awareness of the risks of asbestos and the diseases it causes, and to fund medical research.

As a mesothelioma patient, or as a family member of a patient, you should stay informed regarding these political debates. Listed in the resources section after Question 100 are several books and web sites that provide good background information about asbestos and the politics of asbestos diseases, as well as current information regarding legislative efforts related to asbestos. If you are a union member, union publications and web sites may also be good sources of legal and legislative information.

25. I'm finding more and more people whose lives have been affected by mesothelioma. We all agree that we want to do something about this disease. What can be done at the community level?

Families in a number of states, including Pennsylvania, Minnesota, Montana, California, and Michigan, are working together to increase awareness regarding the health risks of asbestos and the diseases it causes, to raise funds for medical research, and to ensure that the needs and rights of patients and their families are addressed in state and federal legislation.

Working together, families in Pittsburgh, Duluth, and Ann Arbor have raised both asbestos awareness within the community and medical research dollars. More importantly, their efforts have created a community of support and friendship for patients and their families dealing with the reality of mesothelioma. Having the opportunity to talk with others living with the disease has decreased the isolation and fear this disease creates.

The staff and volunteers of the Mesothelioma Applied Research Foundation (Meso Foundation, www.curemeso.org) will gladly assist anyone interested in forming support organizations, raising funds for research, and increasing awareness.

Moreover, it is important to support and thank government officials, whether they are OSHA or EPA staff or members of Congress or your state legislature, who advocate for mesothelioma patients and their families and who work to ensure fair and proactive measures to eradicate this disease and to address the medical and personal well-being of patients. Enormous pressure is exerted on these public servants regularly aimed at eroding patient and family rights.

Contact your local or area American Cancer Society chapter and medical facilities. Identify yourself as someone who is dealing firsthand with mesothelioma. Ask to be listed as a contact for others who may be dealing with this disease.

Write letters to the editor when issues surface regarding asbestos. Do what you can to inform the public that asbestos has not been banned and that even brief exposure to asbestos can seriously affect one's health.

Encourage family members and friends to join you in your efforts to increase community awareness and to influence the legislative process.

26. As someone who's been diagnosed with mesothelioma, do I and my family have any legal rights?

Yes. Because mesothelioma is caused by exposure to asbestos, you may be able to recover medical costs and lost income, as well as personal damages from the asbestos manufacturer(s) if you were exposed in the course of doing your job.

Sue adds . . .

Bruce was hesitant at first to consider litigation. However, after learning more about mesothelioma and asbestos, he realized that litigation is an important step in changing behaviors and actions. Bruce was also a strong advocate for the rights of working people and for justice when one has been wronged. Such litigation is inherent in those rights and in finding justice.

27. How do I learn more about my legal rights?

Contacting an attorney or law firm that specializes in personal injury is the best first step, and legal professionals who have experience in dealing with asbestos-related personal injury are especially helpful. Your primary focus will be on medical issues, and having an attorney who can proceed with what needs to be done legally will be a great source of relief and support for you and your family.

28. How do I find a qualified and reputable attorney?

Good sources of referrals include your doctors, your union if you are or were a union member, your local or state bar association, and other mesothelioma patients and their families. Several of the web sites listed in the resources section after Question 100 may also be able to assist you in finding an attorney.

29. Because of the intensity of dealing with the diagnosis, shouldn't I wait with the legal issues and focus first on medical treatments and recovery?

While that would certainly be ideal, mesothelioma is an unpredictable disease. The information you possess regarding your exposure, including names, dates, and locations, needs to be documented promptly.

Considerable research and follow-up is needed for the attorneys to prepare your case. The earlier you make that initial contact and begin the legal process, the better. Attorneys who specialize in mesothelioma-related personal injury cases are very aware of the physical and emotional stresses of the disease and treatments. They will be sensitive and thoughtful in their work on your case, including scheduling meetings, phone conversations, detailing your exposure, and so on.

30. If my case of mesothelioma is due to work-related exposure, am I eligible for workers' compensation?

Perhaps. Your eligibility will depend on the workers' compensation laws in your state. Your attorney can assist you with your workers' compensation questions.

31. What types of records might be needed for the legal process?

For work-related exposure, you'll need W-2s and other tax records; social security records; and the names, addresses, and phone numbers of work colleagues. For exposure during military service, you'll need your military records. For other types of exposure, the information needed may include the addresses of the site(s) where exposure occurred, the names of others who may be familiar with the exposure, and any known products.

32. Do I need to have a will?

Because of the nature of mesothelioma as well as the injury litigation process, a will is strongly recommended. The timing and size of awards and/or settlements of cases are difficult to predict. Having a will that lays out for your loved ones how you wish to have your assets disbursed well in advance will relieve much stress and anxiety for you and for them. An attorney who specializes in wills and estates can assist you and your family in making wise and timely decisions.

The Politics of Mesothelioma

PART FIVE

Treatment

What is staging, and why is it important?

What is my prognosis?

What are the survival rates for mesothelioma?

What is supportive care in mesothelioma?

What surgery is performed for mesothelioma?

More . . .

33. I have been successful in being referred to a mesothelioma treatment center. What can I expect now?

There should be a "point person" that you have been referred to who is going to be your advocate as your mesothelioma treating physician. This is usually the person who is the expert on site for the disease and is either a medical oncologist, a surgeon, or a radiation oncologist. This individual usually has a track record of performing clinical trials for the disease and may even be involved in laboratory research in the disease. The first visit is going to be a whirlwind; this physician or someone on the staff will be taking a history from you, performing a physical examination, going over all the records you have, looking at your x-rays and CTs, and submitting your slides to the pathologist to give you a second opinion on the diagnosis. There may even be some records or x-rays that fell through the cracks. If this is the case, don't panic! Your physician and the staff at the cancer center will help you secure these missing pieces quickly so the workup will not be delayed.

The first thing your physician advocate should do after meeting you is to educate you about the disease in general terms. You may think of yourself as already being an expert in the disease, but this physician should be able to generalize the issues of mesothelioma and then individualize them to you. All of this sounds like a lot of redundancy. To a certain extent it is, but it leads to the next series of questions that should be answered by this specialist, including the role of staging in mesothelioma, the treatment results, what happens after treatment, and, most importantly to you, a sensitive but realistic discussion of your prognosis with an emphasis on the explosion of treatment options and interest in mesothelioma that is presently occurring.

Sue adds . . .

Remember to keep your notebook handy for all conversations regarding treatment, care instructions, and so on.

34. What is staging, and why is it important?

Staging is a process that attempts to describe the status of the disease at a given moment in time. Staging involves evaluating characteristics of the tumor itself (T), whether the cancer has spread to the lymph nodes (N) or to other parts of the body, known as metastasis (M). Staging is important because it guides the physician in choosing the correct treatment plan for a patient and also gives him or her an idea of what the prognosis may be.

Staging in mesothelioma is, unfortunately, not as clear-cut as in other cancers, because it is such a diffuse disease, and because there are not very many cases on which to standardize a global staging system. There are, in fact, two staging systems, one from the Brigham and Women's Hospital in Boston and another developed by the International Mesothelioma Interest Group (IMIG). Both are similar, but there are subtle differences between the two. Which system is used is not important as long as there is consistency and accuracy in reporting the results of the individual T, N, and M components. In fact, the International Association for the Study of Lung Cancer (IASLC), along with help from worldwide institutions that care for patients with mesothelioma will be revising the staging system sometime in 2009 or 2010.

Basically, as in many other types of cancer, the staging system for mesothelioma consists of four stages. These range from Stage 1, which has the best prognosis, to Stage 4, which means that the cancer has spread to other parts of the body. This stage has the worst prognosis. The staging system is further broken down into the T stage, the N stage, and the M stage. The T stage describes the size of the tumor and evaluates whether the cancer involves nearby important structures. The N stage evaluates the lymph nodes and whether the cancer has spread to nodes inside or outside of the lung. The M stage simply refers to whether the cancer has spread to other parts of the body (or metastasized).

35. What are the staging guidelines for mesothelioma?

Mesothelioma is not like lung cancer, where there is one dominant mass; mesothelioma touches many surfaces, has different thicknesses, and makes it difficult to see whether lymph nodes are involved on the radiographic studies. Clinical staging based on the x-rays and the symptoms in mesothelioma is incredibly difficult. It is really tough for even the experts to say that you have a Stage I or Stage II mesothelioma unless a thoracoscopy has been performed, especially in patients with early stages of the disease. Moreover, even in a case presumed to be in the early stages, the disease could have spread to the lymph nodes, which would make it a Stage III case. In both staging systems, it is recognized that involvement of the **lymph nodes** is important with regard to how long a patient will live. Finally, the IMIG staging system relies on whether the disease has invaded adjacent structures, as opposed to just "sitting on" or "touching" those structures. There are newer ways to try to help with staging including the use of PET scans as mentioned earlier, as well as clinical and laboratory parameters that groups in the United States and Europe use. Some centers are even trying to measure the volume of the disease in order to see if that will give an idea of the true stage.

The bottom line, however, is that the only way to have an absolute accurate staging of these descriptors is via an operation that describes these invasive features and the extent of disease and that takes samples of or removes the lymph nodes for examination.

Although the only accurate way to definitively establish the stage in a patient is "surgical staging," not every patient with mesothelioma should have an operation for treatment. Hence, the "Holy Grail" of future staging for mesothelioma will be when we can just look at the genes or the proteins in the original biopsy specimen and be able to tell our patients their prognosis and how they will do (that is, what their "molecular stage" is) based on these findings. The goal in this situation eventually will be to guide therapy based on these molecular observations.

36. What are lymph nodes?

Lymph nodes are small, bean-shaped structures that are found throughout our body and are part of our immune system. Their function is to trap bacteria and other foreign substances like cancer cells. These nodes cluster in groups and are connected by a system of vessels called **lymphatic vessels**. **Lymph** is a clear, watery liquid made up of excess tissue fluid and protein and is found in the **lymphatic** vessels. The lymph is carried through these vessels to the lymph nodes, where the cells of the immune system can get rid of invading bacteria or other foreign particles. Lymph nodes can enlarge in the presence of an infection as the cells

Treatment

Lymph node (limf node)

A rounded mass of lymphatic tissue that is surrounded by a capsule of connective tissue. Lymph nodes filter lymph (lymphatic fluid), and they store lymphocytes (white blood cells). They are located along lymphatic vessels. Also called a lymph gland. The involvement of lymph glands by mesothelioma changes the stage to a higher one and is an indication of a more advanced tumor.

Lymphatic vessels

Interconnecting tubes that link lymph nodes and allow flow of lymph.

Lymph

Fluid composed of lymphocytes.

Lymphocyte (LIM-fo-site)

A type of white blood cell. Lymphocytes have a number of roles in the immune system, including the production of antibodies and other substances that fight infection and diseases.

within the node (the lymphocytes) increase in number or when tumor cells grow there. This occurs primarily when cancer cells spread from the original site to the lymph nodes. If lymph nodes are found to be enlarged on your CT scans, your doctor may want to evaluate them further by performing a biopsy. This may call for a procedure called a **mediastinoscopy**, which allows a biopsy to be taken of the lymph nodes in the chest. It is a minor operation that requires the use of a special scope. Performing a lymph node biopsy can tell your doctor whether the lymph nodes have cancer in them or are enlarged because of inflammation (swelling) associated with cancer. It is unusual to perform mediastinoscopies in patients with mesothelioma; however, if the lymph nodes that are involved with the tumor are in the opposite side of the chest or outside the area of the chest with the main disease, surgery would not be helpful to you, and this important information would move you to a chemotherapy program as your first treatment. There are some new technologies using ultrasound guided catheters on the end of scopes that are placed in the esophagus and/or the breathing tubes that may be used with increasing frequency to stage the lymph nodes in mesothelioma.

Mediastinoscopy (MEE-dee-a-stin-AHS-ko-pee)

A procedure in which a tube is inserted into the chest to view the organs in the area between the lungs and nearby lymph nodes. The tube is inserted through an incision above the breastbone. This procedure is usually performed to get a tissue sample from the lymph nodes on the right side of the chest.

37. How does mesothelioma spread?

The majority of patients who die of mesothelioma, treated or untreated, will die of complications of the growth of the disease in the cavity (abdomen or chest) it originated in and not from disease that has spread to other parts of the body. The fluid or liquid that is found in the chest will eventually be replaced by a growing solid tumor. This can lead to breathing difficulties, pneumonia, or decreased heart function with arrhythmias (funny irregular heartbeats). This increase in solid mass can also lead to severe pain in the chest wall, requiring narcotic medications. Loss of weight because of poor appetite can also occur. The disease may spread to other areas of the body, but this usually occurs late in the course of the disease. The most frequently involved organs are the liver, the adrenal gland, the kidney, and the opposite lung.

38. What is my prognosis?

In general, your prognosis depends on the following factors: the size of the cancer, how extensively it has spread, how the cancer looks under the microscope, and how the cancer responds to treatment. Although the overall prognosis for patients with mesothelioma is poor, some patients live with the disease for a considerable period of time. There are some factors that have been found to predict which patients will do better than others, including the type of mesothelioma that is present, how much solid tumor is present, and the functional status of the patient. Functional status is defined as an individual's ability to perform daily activities required to fulfill basic needs, perform usual roles, and maintain health and well-being. The better functional ability you have the better prognosis. Women tend to do better than men. If you have the epithelial type of mesothelioma as opposed to the other two types, you also have an advantage. The more functional ability you have (the ability to do normal tasks of daily living), the better the prognosis. The age at which you are diagnosed is also important, because the older you are the worse you tend to do. Lastly, there are certain blood values that tend to indicate who will have a worse prognosis. If the platelet cell count (cells that are responsible for making blood clot) is elevated, the hemoglobin (cells that carry oxygen) is low, and the white blood cells (cells that fight infection) are high, these abnormal blood values may indicate a poorer prognosis.

39. What are the survival rates for mesothelioma?

The estimated survival rate for patients who choose to have only supportive care (treatment directed at controlling symptoms) ranges from four to nine months. Approximately 50% of patients die within six months if no treatment other than supportive care is given. Patients who meet the criteria to be enrolled in clinical trials that use multiple treatments (multimodal trials, described later), tend to survive longer, and 50% of these patients live 8 to 18 months after treatment. As a patient, however, you must realize that you are an individual case, and there are many subsets that add up to these statistics. For example, if you were diagnosed very early, and have disease only on the parietal pleura, your chance for survival is much better, with 70% of the patients living for five years. However, once the disease involves the lung without invading it (although still Stage I if the lymph nodes are not involved), the survival rate decreases to a 30% chance of living for five years.

40. What do these scary survival rates mean to me as a patient?

Your doctor is only being frank with you when he discusses these survival rates. You may be a candidate for therapies that are different from the older therapies that generated these statistics. These are also only general statistics in small numbers of patients, and your treatment will probably be very different from these older results in the literature. It is important to remember that the treatment for mesothelioma is rapidly changing, and we are learning much more about this disease at an incredibly accelerated rate. As a patient you are going to have to remind yourself that you are a new explorer as part of a mission to eradicate the disease. You may participate in options that your physicians have great hopes for, but for which they might not be able to forecast the future.

41. What is supportive care in mesothelioma?

The best treatment options for patients with mesothelioma are constantly under study; however, there are currently much fewer "standards of care" for doctors to follow, as there are for other types of cancer, such as lung cancer. Much still needs to be learned about the disease, and that is why your doctor must explain the newest clinical protocols for the disease (see the next question). Treatment decisions are frequently based on how well the patient can function from day to day and what the treating physician's knowledge and attitudes are about the disease. As I discussed previously, some doctors may not see this disease very often and may not be aware of new types of treatments that are available in other areas of the country, or they may feel that the standard of care should be treatment of symptoms only (supportive care). You have already read that the median survival of patients who receive this type of supportive care ranges from four to nine months. Therefore, this type of treatment is usually reserved for those people who refuse or are not candidates for a more aggressive treatment plan.

What symptoms can be made better without attempting to treat the cancer? The most common symptom of this disease is shortness of breath caused by a recurring buildup of fluid in the chest or abdomen. Unfortunately, this sometimes causes a quick reaction by the doctor to perform a procedure to get rid of the fluid. This procedure is called a **pleurodesis** and involves putting a medication (usually talc, a mineral in loose form also known as talcum powder), into the pleural

Pleurodesis (PLOO-ro-DEE-sis)

A medical procedure that uses chemicals or drugs to cause inflammation and adhesion between the layers of the pleura (the tissue that covers the lungs and lines the interior wall of the chest cavity). This prevents the buildup of fluid in the pleural cavity. It is used as a treatment for severe pleural effusion. Can be performed with a variety of agents.

space (the space between the chest wall and lung) to cause the visceral pleura (the lining on the lung) and the parietal pleura (the lining on the chest wall) to stick to each other. This gets rid of the space so fluid can no longer accumulate there. The problem with this procedure is that it can interfere with other potential treatment options and make surgery more difficult. The fluid can no longer accumulate in the pleural space but will eventually be replaced by a bulky solid mass due to its natural history and the way it spreads. Nevertheless, control of the fluid is important for those patients who are not candidates or who refuse the more aggressive approaches.

Other supportive care measures include the insertion of a PleurX catheter (a thin chest catheter) into the pleural space that allows drainage of the fluid as it builds up. Patients and their care providers are taught how to drain these catheters at home, which allows more freedom for the patient. It is also an effective way of managing recurring fluid problems. Although at first draining the fluid may be a bit unnerving, it is a convenient and safe way to keep the patient comfortable without added trips to and from the clinic or hospital.

Multimodality treatment

Therapy that combines more than one method of treatment.

Chest pain is another symptom that requires intervention by the health care team. Treatment may include narcotic medications or surgical blocks (a nerve block relieves pain by injecting a substance into or around a nerve and is used when pain affects a small region of your body) or pump insertions to control pain.

42. What, in general, are the non-supportive care treatment options in mesothelioma?

Patients with mesothelioma should understand that they can be treated with many treatments together that could work better than single treatments alone but may be associated with more complications or toxicities. These **multimodal** approaches are more aggressive than single treatment options. Aggressive treatment approaches for mesothelioma involve the use of surgery (taking out as much of the cancer as possible) as part of the treatment package. The surgery may be combined with chemotherapy (medications to kill cancer cells) and radiation therapy (use of high-dose x-rays to kill the cancer cells). If surgery is to be considered, a patient must have a complete workup beforehand, to help assess his or her level of functioning and ability to handle the surgery. Question 45 discusses what a workup involves.

The purpose of the surgery is to remove as much of the cancer as possible, down to a level that is not detected by the human eye; however, not all of the cancer can be removed at the time of the operation because this disease spreads across all the surfaces in the chest and floats around these areas. Therefore, surgeons can never be sure that they have gotten rid of every cell or, as is described in the literature "established negative margins." This is the reason that surgery should be combined with another form of treatment, either before, during, or after the operation, so that these other invisible cells that are circulating can potentially be killed.

Many treatment combinations are currently being studied. Those that combine surgery, chemotherapy, and radiation may give the best results. Sometimes chemotherapy is given before surgery to try to shrink the tumor. Surgery is then performed, and afterwards patients receive either more chemotherapy or radiation therapy. This approach has been used in selected patients since 2000, and has been validated as feasible and promising in trials not only in the United States but also in Europe. In general, radiation is given only to those who have had the lung and pleura removed (extrapleural pneumonectomy, removal of the lung, more details to follow) since there is no concern about damaging the lung, as it has been removed already. New ways of giving radiation, however, are also being studied to see how effective they are and to see if the areas of treatment can spare the lungs. This type of radiation therapy is called intensity modulation radiation therapy (IMRT). Radiation therapy is never given alone as a primary treatment but is used only in combination with surgery and/or chemotherapy. This is because the large doses of radiation that are needed to potentially cure the disease carry the risk of severely damaging the normal tissues.

If a patient is unable to receive or chooses not to have surgery, he or she may receive chemotherapy alone. The effectiveness of the chemotherapy drugs that have been available in the past was poor. With the development of new agents, however, tumor response to chemotherapy has improved, but we are not satisfied despite the doubling of response rates, and even newer agents and combinations are being studied.

43. What is performance status, and why is it important?

Performance status is a measurement of a person's overall state of health. It is a very important measure to look at because it helps the doctor decide whether a patient is fit enough to receive treatment for cancer. It also gives an indication of how well a person might tolerate a particular type of therapy. Two types of scales are used to evaluate **performance status**, and

Performance status
A measure of how well a patient is able to perform ordinary tasks and carry out daily activities.

although they look different the end goal is the same. These scales are also used to evaluate patients for their ability to be treated in research protocols or studies (clinical trials) that look at and try to answer specific treatment questions. Both scales use a rating from 1 to 4 with 1 being those patients with no symptoms at all who can perform all normal activities. A performance status of 4 is the worst category, as those that are in this group are mostly bedridden.

44. What surgery is performed for mesothelioma?

There are, in general, three types of operations or surgical procedures that may be performed on patients with mesothelioma. These include thoracoscopy, **pleurectomy/ decortication**, and **extrapleural pneumonectomy** (EPP). As we mentioned earlier, a thoracoscopy (the use of a scope to look inside the chest) is usually performed in order to get a diagnosis of mesothelioma or to help treat shortness of breath by removing fluid in the pleural space. The second type of surgery is called a pleurectomy/decortication. This procedure involves the removal of the linings in the chest or abdomen. The last type is called an extrapleural pneumonectomy (EPP) and involves the removal of the lung and the pleura on the affected side. In a majority of the cases, part or all of the diaphragm is also removed, as well as the pericardial sac. This is a complex operation that should be performed only by skilled surgeons who have experience with the disease.

45. What determines whether I am able to have surgery?

Before any surgery is attempted, you must have a complete **workup** to assess how functional you are and whether you would be able to tolerate surgery. During

Pleurectomy/ decortication

An operation for mesothelioma that removes the involved pleura and frees the underlying lung so that it can expand and fill the pleural cavity.

Extrapleural pneumonectomy

Surgery to remove a diseased lung, part of the pericardium (membrane covering the heart), part of the diaphragm (muscle between the lungs and the abdomen), and part of the parietal pleura (membrane lining the chest). This type of surgery is used most often to treat malignant mesothelioma.

Workup

A series of tests to discover information about the patient, most commonly to define extent of disease or suitability for a given treatment.

a workup, a number of routine tests are performed, including an assessment of lung and heart function. Patients being considered for surgery need to have disease on only one side of the chest or, in cases of peritoneal mesothelioma, the disease must be contained within the abdomen. The disease must not have spread anywhere else. They also need to have a good performance status with few symptoms of their disease. This would put them in a category or performance status of 0 or 1. They need to have good lung function with adequate lung reserve so that after the surgery they are still able to perform their normal activities. Lastly, their heart must be in good shape and able to withstand a lengthy surgical procedure.

46. What determines which surgical procedure I will have?

The operation that is chosen depends upon the extent of the disease, your level of functioning, including your overall health status, the attitudes of the treating institution, and, if you are participating in a protocol, the surgery that the protocol calls for. Basically, there are three categories to consider before one procedure is chosen over the other. Is the surgery being performed (1) to control symptoms, (2) as part of combination therapy, or (3) to deliver new types of therapies in the operating room?

There are no real guidelines before surgery that a doctor can use to assure patients as to what operation will be necessary to remove as much of the tumor as possible. A CT scan can help guide the physician, but the real test is in the operating room, where the surgeon can actually see and assess the area better. The attitude of the individual surgeon can also play a role in the choice of operation performed. Some surgeons save an EPP for those patients with bulky tumors that prevent a simple pleurectomy from being performed. This saves the patient from having a lung removed and all the other problems that can arise as a result. Others feel that the greatest chance for complete removal of as much tumor as possible is with an EPP even in patients with minimal disease. For surgeons who do not feel that the only operation to perform to remove the disease is an EPP, the final decision as to whether a pleurectomy/decortication or EPP is performed is sometimes made in the operating room unless a patient is in a clinical trial that calls specifically for one operation or another.

The argument over what is the best surgical procedure remains one of the most controversial and emotionally debated aspects of the treatment of mesothelioma. The decision making becomes even more controversial in cases of early mesothelioma where there is minimal or no involvement of the lung and the disease is primarily on the parietal pleura. All thoracic surgeons have agreed that performing an EPP for any reason can have long-term health implications for the patient, and unfortunately there are no data specifically comparing one operation to another in this disease for patients with the same early stage.

Another complicating issue is the use of talc and other material placed into the chest when a diagnosis is made in order to prevent further fluid accumulation. A common scenario occurs when the patient has a lot of fluid but minimal solid tumor, most of it is on the inner lining of the chest. If that patient has a talc or other material added to the chest cavity, cementing the lung to the chest wall, it may severely affect the chance for an EPP.

The bottom line is that the patient, understanding the controversy of this question, must not be a silent witness to these discussions. The patient must understand how much disease he or she has, whether an EPP is indeed feasible, whether a protocol he or she intends to enroll in demands a certain type of surgery, the chances of recurrence with either operation, and finally the attitude of the surgeon. It is not unheard of for patients to "call the shots" in nonprotocol situations and say that the surgeon should not perform an EPP even if a situation in the operating room demands one. This is a very unusual occurrence and leaves an inordinate burden on the patient. Such issues illustrate why establishing a relationship with your "treatment team" from the very beginning, in which you get a feeling of trust, caring, and expertise, will not lead to regrets after all is said and done.

47. What can I expect before surgery, and what can I do to prepare for it?

You will be scheduled for certain tests prior to your surgery that will help to evaluate your readiness for the procedure. Your doctor will let you know what tests are needed and where they will be performed. Appointment times and dates for these tests will also be given to you. It is important not to miss any scheduled appointments, as this may delay your surgery.

Patients may want to donate their own blood for the surgery, and family members may wish to donate blood. This can be arranged through the hospital's blood bank in conjunction with the local Red Cross. You are able to donate one or more units of blood that can then be banked for you until your surgery. There is a time limit for completing the donation and for how long blood can be stored after it is collected. For this reason it is important to call and find out the details as soon as you make the decision to donate.

Your nutritional state can also affect your surgical risk. Prior to surgery it is necessary to eat as well as possible and to include high-protein and high-calorie foods in your diet. You should try to avoid losing any weight during this time period. Ask to speak to a dietician if you need assistance in this area. Let your doctor know if you are currently taking any medications to thin your blood, including aspirin, Plavix, Coumadin, and non-steroidal anti-inflammatory medications. You will need to stop taking these prior to surgery, and your doctor can give you specific instructions on this. You will have preoperative (before surgery) testing done approximately three days before your surgery. At that time you will have routine blood work, an EKG, and a chest x-ray, and you will also be seen by an anesthesiologist (a doctor responsible for administering the medications that will put you to sleep during the operation). During this visit you will also be given specific instructions about the surgery itself. Finally, if you are a smoker, you need to stop!

48. What tests will I need before surgery to define what procedure I can tolerate?

The majority of patients who receive surgery for mesothelioma are middle-aged to older individuals. For this reason it is important that a thorough heart evaluation be performed, especially if there has been a history of heart problems in the past. This should include an echocardiogram (ultrasound of the heart) as well as an evaluation by a cardiologist or heart doctor. It is the responsibility of the cardiologist and the surgeon to make sure your heart can withstand surgery. They may want to conduct further tests on you to make sure your heart is functioning properly, which may include a stress test of your heart. The cardiologist will then let your surgeon know the results and whether or not you have been cleared for the surgery.

The other tests that are usually performed are related to your lungs and how well they function. Your right lung normally contributes 55% of the function and the left lung 45%. Before knowing whether a patient is a candidate for an EPP, it is a good idea to tell him or her what to expect if a lung is removed. A pulmonary function test and a quantitative lung perfusion scan are routinely performed to accomplish this goal. The perfusion scan assigns numbers to regions of the lung so that the surgeon can estimate the residual amount of lung that will be left after the operation. The doctor will be able to assess whether oxygen will be required after surgery and for how long. He or she will also be able to predict how the surgery may affect your ability to do what you normally do. These are all very important considerations that may determine whether or not you are able (or want!) to have surgery.

49. What should I expect following my surgery? What are the common complications of surgery for mesothelioma?

Whether you have a pleurectomy/decortication or an EPP, both are major endeavors. Recovery time will vary with each individual, but the average time it takes to regain your strength and energy is usually four to six weeks. Unfortunately, there is always some pain and discomfort after surgery. At the majority of centers performing these operations, patients receive an epidural catheter that is put in at the time of the operation. This catheter is inserted into the spine while you are asleep, and numbing medication is put into the catheter. This medication puts the whole chest to sleep temporarily after the operation. You can then cough and breathe deeply more easily, which helps decrease the chance of infection and other complications. The epidural catheter remains in place for three days and is then removed. After it is removed, you will be switched to an oral (by mouth) narcotic pain medication, which helps to control the pain. You will continue to take this pain medication even after you are discharged and sent home. Gradually, over the next few weeks, your need for pain medications will decrease and you may be weaned off the narcotics and onto other forms of pain medicine that are not as strong, or you may not need to take any pain medication at all.

Chest tubes are also inserted during surgery. These small, flexible tubes will be present when you awake and will remain in place for approximately three days after surgery. The purpose of the tubes is to drain fluid and air that have collected in the chest due to the surgery.

Empyema
Infected fluid (pus) in the chest which can result postoperatively as a complication of surgery for mesothelioma.

You may feel short of breath after surgery and may require oxygen temporarily. Breathing does improve over time, and the need for oxygen will also decrease as you get further out from the surgery.

When pleurectomy/decortications are performed routinely for mesothelioma, few major complications are usually seen. Allowing the lungs to heal after stripping the pleura from them may require the chest tubes to remain in for longer than usual, sometimes up to 10 days. Pneumonia and respiratory problems may occur and are usually related to the size of the mass removed and a decreased level of functioning before the operation.

Hemorrhage

In medicine, loss of blood from damaged blood vessels. A hemorrhage may be internal or external, and usually involves a lot of bleeding in a short time.

Arrhythmia

An arrhythmia is any deviation from or disturbance of the normal heart rhythm.

Bronchopleural fistula

A complication after extrapleural pneumonectomy in which there is a leakage of air from the closed bronchial tube.

Pulmonary embolism

Migration of a clot, usually from the legs, to the heart resulting in the blockage of arteries to the lung and resulting in acute shortness of breath. A possible cause of morbidity and morality from operations for mesothelioma.

Empyema (the accumulation of pus in the chest) is rare and is managed by longer chest tube drainage and antibiotics. **Hemorrhage** or bleeding that requires a doctor to open the chest back up to find the cause and correct it is very rare.

Due to the size and magnitude of the operation, an EPP has more risk of complications than a pleurectomy. The most common complication is an **arrhythmia,** which is usually a fast, irregular heartbeat. These occur because the heart is being manipulated during surgery and becomes irritated. The treatment for an arrhythmia involves starting the patient on specific heart medications. Patients are usually kept on these medications for about one month after surgery, and then they can be stopped. The most feared complication after an EPP is when the breathing tube to the lung that has been removed develops an opening and air is coming into an empty chest. Fluid also drains through this hole to the opposite lung. This is known as a **bronchopleural fistula** and may require a second operation to repair the opening, or external drainage with later repair if the problem occurs at some time after the original operation. The most common symptom of a bronchopleural fistula is a persistent cough, so if a cough develops make sure to inform your surgeon. This complication can lead to pulmonary failure, pneumonia, and death. Recognized early, however, it can be treated successfully.

Heart attack, as well as a clot going to the remaining lung from the legs (**pulmonary embolism**) are also risks after an EPP. Finally, unusual but dramatic complications can include the heart falling through an opening in the newly constructed pericardium (hernia), or failure of the newly constructed diaphragm to keep the abdominal contents out of the chest (chiefly on the left side). These reconstructions are performed with foreign material, usually Gortex, and there is a remote chance that they can become infected and need to be removed. Rapid accumulation of fluid in the chest once you start eating, or a change in the color of the chest tube drainage to a grayish, pussy color could mean that the tube carrying lymph from the belly through the chest has been injured. In cases of EPPs, this situation may call for a second operation to close the leak, while with pleurectomies, continued drainage and changing the patient's diet may allow this to close.

Sue adds . . .

Bruce's recovery from surgery was relatively complication free. He went home six days after his surgery and was taking brief walks near our home within two weeks. A few weeks later, he returned to work. He was cautious about not overextending himself but was grateful to return to a daily routine that provided a distraction from the diagnosis.

50. What is chemotherapy? How does it work?

Chemotherapy is a general term to describe the use of chemicals or medications to treat disease, especially cancer. It's the treatment of cancer with a special group of drugs that are able to destroy cancer cells. There are many types of chemotherapy drugs, and each has a different way of attacking the cancer cells. In cancer treatment these medications can be used alone, but are more often used in combination with each other, to get the best overall effect. This is because studies have shown that these drugs work better when they are used with other types of chemotherapy agents than they do when given by themselves. Chemotherapy is considered the "systemic" treatment for mesothelioma because it is able to go to most parts of the body through the bloodstream. This means that chemotherapy is able to travel through the body looking for any cancer cells that may have broken away from the original tumor.

Normal cells in the body grow and then die in a very precise and controlled fashion. Cancer cells, however, continue to grow, divide and multiply uncontrollably. Chemotherapy interferes with this growth and stops cancer cells from reproducing at certain points in their life cycle. This, in turn, kills these abnormal cancer cells but also affects normal cells at the same time. The reason that this happens is that anticancer drugs act on any cells in the body that divide rapidly, not just cancer cells. The types of cells that are most likely to be affected include those found in the gastrointestinal (GI) tract, bone marrow, hair follicles and reproductive system. This is the cause of many of the side effects that are commonly seen during chemotherapy treatment.

Adjuvant therapy (AD-joo-vant)
Treatment given after the primary treatment to increase the chances of a cure. Adjuvant therapy may include chemotherapy, radiation therapy, hormone therapy, or biological therapy.

Chemotherapy can be given by itself as the primary type of treatment to help keep the cancer from spreading, to shrink the tumor, or to relieve symptoms. It may also cure cancer in some types of tumors. It is more common, however, to see chemotherapy combined with other forms of treatment like surgery and radiation. In some instances, chemotherapy can be used before surgery to help shrink the tumor and make the surgery easier to perform. It may also be used after surgery, to help get rid of any cancer cells that may be left behind that are too small to see. When chemotherapy is used in this way it is called **adjuvant therapy**.

51. What can I expect during chemotherapy? How many treatments will I need?

Your doctor will decide which chemotherapy drugs you will receive. Chemotherapy can be given in a number of places, and the choice depends on the types of drugs ordered, the policies of the hospital, and what your doctor prefers. It can be given in a clinic, in your hospital's outpatient department, or in a hospital. If you receive chemotherapy in the hospital, you may have to stay overnight so that the doctor can watch you closely. He or she will watch you for any side effects that might occur from the medications you will receive and make changes as necessary. Chemotherapy drugs can be given by mouth, through a vein, or directly into an organ or body cavity.

The chemotherapy you will receive will most likely be administered directly into your vein (IV or intravenously), through a thin needle or catheter that allows the drug to enter right into your bloodstream. Having the needle placed for an IV feels the same as having blood drawn for a blood test. The difference is that during chemotherapy the needle remains in place for a longer period of time. Sometimes you may feel a cool sensation or slight burning at the insertion site when the actual IV is started. If you notice any burning, pain, or discomfort during or after an IV treatment, let your nurse or doctor know right away. Some drugs may cause redness and damage to the tissue if they leak out of the vein. A more permanent type of catheter may be necessary if a person has any type of problem or if it becomes difficult to insert the needle into a vein for each treatment. A doctor will insert this catheter into a large vein, and it will remain in place throughout your whole course of treatment. There are different types of catheters that are used for this purpose. Your doctor will explain to you which catheter he or she is going to put in and what you need to do to take care of it.

You should always let your doctor know what medications you are taking before you start treatment. Some medications should not be taken while you are receiving chemotherapy because they may interfere with the effects of the drug. Remember to report even over-the-counter drugs like vitamins and cold pills. Your doctor will let you know if you should stop taking any of them. After your treatment begins, let your doctor know of any changes in your medications, and check with him or her before starting anything new.

Your doctor will decide how many treatments of chemotherapy you will receive, the specific doses, and how often they will be given. The choice depends on the drugs that are being used and how your body responds to them. You may receive treatment every day, once a week, or every few weeks. It is often given with rest periods in between doses so that your body has a chance to recover from the effects of treatment and build healthy new cells. This break also helps you to regain some strength before beginning the next chemotherapy cycle or session. The chemotherapy schedule is typically outlined in cycles (one treatment), with the rest periods between the cycles. A course of chemotherapy is the cycles in your entire treatment plan. Cycle lengths may vary, but a typical chemotherapy course consists of multiple cycles. In most cases you will receive approximately two or three cycles of the drugs and then be reevaluated with CT scans to see if your cancer is responding to the treatment. The doctor will then decide what the next step in the plan will be. It is important to follow the schedule that your doctor lays out for you so that you can receive the desired effect from the chemotherapy. If you miss or are unable to make a treatment session, contact your doctor immediately so that you can receive instructions about what to do.

52. Why are blood tests ordered during my chemotherapy treatment? What are blood counts, and what should I know about them?

There are many side effects of chemotherapy that you might experience. Cancer cells grow and divide rapidly, and chemotherapy drugs are aimed at killing these types of cells. Unfortunately, they also harm healthy cells that divide rapidly. There are 3 major types of blood cells located in the bone marrow (where blood cells are produced). As with all cells in the body, each blood cell has a specific function and set life expectancy, so they are constantly replaced by new cells made by the bone marrow. A common side effect of chemotherapy is that it damages healthy bone marrow cells, and causes a temporary shortage of the healthy, replacement cells. The 3 major types of blood cells include white blood cells (cells that help to fight infection), red blood cells (cells that carry oxygen to other parts of the body), and platelets (cells that cause the blood to clot). Blood tests are ordered each week to check the levels of each of these types of blood cells, to make sure they are at an acceptable level in the bloodstream.

The effect chemotherapy has on the bone marrow can drastically lower the number of white blood cells that are available to help your body fight off infection. Your risk of getting an infection is much higher when these cells are low. Infections can occur in almost any part of the body, including the lungs, urinary tract, rectum, and mouth, to name a few. If your white blood cell count (WBC) falls too low, your doctor may decide to delay your next treatment, prescribe medication that can help your bone marrow make new white blood cells, or give you a lower dose of chemotherapy to give these cells a chance to recover.

Chemotherapy can also cause a decrease in the number of red blood cells, which help deliver oxygen to the tissues in the body. If these cells are decreased, the tissues may not be getting enough oxygen to do what they need to do. This is also known as anemia and can cause a person to feel extremely tired. It can also cause dizziness, shortness of breath, feeling cold or weak. If your red blood cell count (RBC) becomes too low, you may need medication that can help your bone marrow make new red blood cells or a blood transfusion before continuing with treatment. This will increase the number of red blood cells in your body.

Lastly, the number of platelets in your bloodstream may be decreased because of your treatment and its effect on the bone marrow. Platelets help stop bleeding by causing the blood to clot. You may notice that you bleed or bruise more easily when your platelets are low. If your platelet count becomes too low, your doctor may give you a transfusion of platelets. Because of the risk of low platelets during chemotherapy, it's important to notify your health care team if you notice any bleeding from the nose or the gums, red spots on the skin, unexpected bruising, or bloody bowel movements.

It is very important that your doctor monitor these blood cell counts frequently by ordering a complete blood cell count (CBC) and platelet count as part of your blood work.

53. What are the common side effects of chemotherapy?

Most people have questions and concerns about the side effects of chemotherapy. They wonder what types of side effects may occur and how to best cope with them if they do. They have often heard horror stories of others' experiences and are frightened that they will have the same difficulties. Now, with the newer chemotherapy drugs that are available, as well as the improvement in the drugs that decrease or prevent nausea and vomiting, treatment is much more tolerable than in the past. It is often overwhelming to hear the wide range of possible side effects associated with these drugs. There are two general rules to understand about side effects. First, no one drug will cause every side effect listed, each drug has a specific profile of side effects due to the unique way it attacks the cancer cells. Second, it is important to remember is that these effects vary from one person to another. Not everyone receiving chemotherapy will experience all or even most of these side effects, and some people have very few, if any. The type and severity of side effects that you will have are related to the type of chemotherapy you receive and the way your body handles the treatment. If you do experience a particular side effect after your initial treatment, you may not experience it the next time you receive the drug. Before starting chemotherapy you should discuss with your doctor and nurse the types of side effects that are most likely to occur, how long they are expected to last, and when you should call the doctor.

There are a few side effects that are commonly seen in people receiving chemotherapy. These include fatigue, nausea and vomiting, and hair loss. Other effects that can occur include constipation, diarrhea, blood clots, decreased blood counts, and neuropathies (loss of sensation and/or tingling in the hands and feet). These occur because normal, rapidly growing cells in the digestive tract, reproductive system, bone marrow, and hair follicles can be damaged by anticancer drugs. Some side effects are minor and annoying, while others can be severe. If severe, they may prevent you from receiving your chemotherapy as the doctor originally planned. This can cause delays in your treatment.

After you have received all of your chemotherapy and your normal cells have had a chance to recover, most of the side effects you experienced will gradually disappear. Some of them will go away quickly while others may take months. Occasionally, some can cause permanent damage. Side effects can be discouraging and bothersome, but they must be compared and weighed against the chemotherapy's ability to kill the cancer cells. Let your doctor or nurse know of any difficulties you are experiencing so he or she can offer suggestions on how to manage these side effects.

Sue adds . . .

Bruce experienced a significant change in his appetite. Foods he previously enjoyed were too salty or too spicy. We altered the "menu" to include a little more comfort food and a lot less seasonings and spices. Drinking lots of water—without ice—helped relieve some of the nausea and aftertaste.

54. What is radiation therapy?

Radiation therapy is a type of cancer treatment that can be used in combination with other therapies such as chemotherapy and surgery. It can also be used alone to treat symptoms that are caused by the cancer. Other names for radiation therapy include irradiation, radiotherapy, cobalt treatment, and x-ray therapy. Special cancer doctors, called radiation oncologists, are responsible for providing this type of treatment. They will work with your doctor to decide the type, amount, and frequency of your treatment with radiation. If you are to receive radiation therapy, you will have a meeting with the radiation oncologist beforehand to discuss the treatment plan.

55. How does radiation work?

Radiation therapy uses high-energy rays to kill cancer cells. Doctors first discovered that they could use radiation (x-rays) to help them see inside the human body and locate disease. Soon after, they discovered that these same rays could be used to treat disease as well. These rays are carefully directed at tumors for brief periods and cause the cancer cells to become injured. This prevents the cancer cells from growing and dividing, which in turn kills the cells and slows down or stops the growth of the tumor. Unfortunately, normal cells in the treatment area are also affected by this radiation but are able to recover quickly.

56. What is a dose of radiation, and how many treatments will I need?

The radiation treatment plan that is recommended for you will depend on the type of cancer you have, your general health, your test results, and the other treatment you are receiving. The first stage of treatment is called the planning stage or simulation. At this time the radiation oncologist will decide the exact location of treatment, the total dose of radiation that you will need, and the number of treatments required. The total dose of radiation is divided into daily doses called fractionations. This is to ensure that it does its intended job with the least amount of damage to your normal cells. The number of radiation treatments required will vary depending on your individual situation. Radiation treatments are usually given five days a week for several weeks, but can also be given daily for a week or more or as a single dose.

Your first visit to the radiation oncologist will be a simulation involving many steps. For this reason it can take hours, so it is important that you plan your day around this appointment. A radiation physicist or dosimetrist helps the radiation oncologist plan the treatment and is also responsible for making sure the treatment machines are functioning properly at all times. You will probably not receive a radiation treatment on this first visit but will be given a daily radiation time and start date before you go home.

The exact place on the body where the high-energy rays will be directed is called the treatment area. A technologist will locate this area using an x-ray machine while you lie still on a table. After the area is located the technologist or doctor will mark your skin with a colored indelible ink marker, creating a tattoo. This must not be washed off the skin until all your treatment has been completed. If for some reason the mark fades or comes off, do not try to draw it back on yourself. Instead, notify your doctor right away. Sometimes a plastic or plaster cast or form of the proposed treatment site has to be made. This form helps you to stay in the same position for each treatment.

57. What equipment is used to deliver radiation?

The type of radiation you will probably receive is called external beam radiation. There are various machines that deliver this kind of radiation to the cancer, including the cobalt machine and the linear accelerator. These machines give the same type of treatment but work in slightly different ways. This equipment is located in either a hospital or a special treatment center, and radiation is usually given as an outpatient treatment.

58. What can I expect during radiation?

Your doctor will be monitoring your progress throughout your radiation treatment. Since radiation affects both cancer cells and normal cells, you will be assessed for any side effects that may occur. Blood tests will be performed, and you will see your doctor for a physical exam on a frequent basis. Alert your doctor or nurse if you notice any side effects so that they can be managed before they become severe. Some people are able to continue doing things that they normally do while undergoing radiation treatment. Others find that they need more rest than usual. Your body is using a lot of extra energy during this time, and you may require more sleep than you normally do. Be sure to listen to your body and rest as often as necessary. If you are receiving external beam radiation, you are not radioactive, and therefore you don't have to limit your contact with others. You do need to avoid anyone with an infection, such as a cold or flu, because your resistance may be lowered while you are undergoing treatment. It is also important to eat well during this time to try to maintain your weight. Communicate with your doctor, nurse, or technologist, and don't be afraid to ask questions.

They are more than willing to help you through your treatment and advise you as necessary.

59. What is the actual radiation procedure like?

When you arrive for your treatment, you will probably be asked to put on a hospital gown. You will then be brought to the treatment room, where you will be assisted onto the treatment table. The radiation therapy technologist will position you and adjust the machines so that everything lines up with the marks on your skin. Special lead shields may be used to protect your normal organs and tissues. They are placed between the machine and the part of your body they are trying to protect. It is very important that you stay as still as possible throughout the entire treatment. Once everything is set up, the technologist will leave the room and turn on the machine. He or she will control the machine from a room nearby and monitor all activities at the same time. Remember, the technologist is able to watch you through a window or on a TV screen during the entire treatment, and you can talk with him or her at any time through a speaker that connects the two rooms. The treatment machines do make noises as they move around your body. They are trying to get at the cancer from different angles and are under the technologist's control at all times. The noise these machines make can sound much like a vacuum cleaner. You should not feel any discomfort at all from the treatment, and you will not see or hear the radiation itself. If you have any fears or are not feeling well during the treatment, let the technologist know immediately.

60. How long does each treatment take?

The actual time required to deliver the radiation itself is very short. It takes only about 1 to 5 minutes to receive the actual treatment dose, even though you can be in the treatment room for around 15 to 20 minutes getting prepared. Delays can happen at any point along the way, so it is important to remember that there may be times when you will have to wait longer than expected for your treatment. Your treatment time is negotiated before treatment starts and usually remains the same throughout your therapy. The radiation team will work with you to develop the best appointment schedule to suit your needs, but please let them know if you are going to be late or miss an appointment. To ensure that you get the most benefit from your treatment, you must receive all ordered doses. Therefore, if you miss an appointment, you will have to make it up at some point before the end of your therapy.

61. What are the common side effects of radiation?

During the course of destroying cancer cells, radiation also damages normal cells that are in the treatment area or field. The end result is the development of side effects. These side effects depend upon the area of the body being treated, the dose given, and the size of the radiation field. Some people don't experience any negative effects from their treatment, while others have very few side effects. If you develop a severe side effect from the radiation, your doctor may want to give you a break from your treatment for a short period. Certain side effects are common no matter what area of the body is being treated. These include fatigue, loss of appetite, and skin reactions or irritations. Other side effects are related to the specific area of the body that is within the treatment field. When receiving radiation to the chest area, you may experience certain side effects, including esophagitis (swelling of the esophagus), fibrosis (the formation of scar tissue), pneumonitis (radiation lung injury), sore throat, and loss of hair in the treated area. Although it can happen, nausea is not commonly seen when receiving chest radiation. Be sure to discuss these specific side effects with your doctor or nurse and report any that occur. He or she will be able to help you deal with them and suggest ways to prevent them in the future.

Sue adds . . .

Bruce received radiation therapy for six weeks, five days a week. Within a few days, he began to experience some of the side effects noted here, most especially fatigue, loss of appetite, and some skin reaction.

PART SIX

Decision Making

What is standard therapy?

What are clinical trials?

What are some experimental investigative treatments for mesothelioma?

More . . .

62. What are the standard treatment options for mesothelioma?

There are currently no published standards of care for the treatment of mesothelioma. Chemotherapy has been used over the years to try to shrink these tumors. However, the problem with the older chemotherapy drugs is that they haven't worked very well. Doctors have now found that it may be best to combine surgery and chemotherapy, using newer drugs in people who are healthy enough to tolerate them. These newer drugs have been found to work better than the drugs used in the past, and combining them with surgery could allow people to live longer.

The First-line (the first chemotherapy treatment used to treat your cancer) chemotherapy agent for mesothelioma is generally a combination of two chemotherapeutic agents, *Cisplatin and Pemetrexed*. Cisplatin is a chemotherapeutic agent, which is the first member of the class of drugs called "alkylating agents" (a group of agents that works by attaching an alkyl agent to the DNA of cells. The theory is that cancer cells are destroyed through this process). Cisplatin is administered intravenously (through a catheter placed in your vein), and there is no oral (by mouth) form. Since Cisplatin is an irritant (can cause inflammation of the veins), it is very important to let your doctor or nurse know if you experience any discomfort at the IV site during, or after, the infusion. The dose of the drug will depend on many factors including your age, height, weight, and general health status. Cisplatin is given over 1 to 2 hours every three weeks.

Cisplatin affects normal cells just like all other chemotherapies, so possible side effects will include low blood cell counts as well as fatigue, nausea, and hair loss, as discussed earlier. There are some specific side effects of Cisplatin, however. The drug can cause damage to the kidneys. For this reason, your doctor will check your baseline kidney function (labs to measure kidney function, before you receive any Cisplatin) to determine if your kidneys are strong enough to process the drug. While you're on Cisplatin therapy there are some actions that can be taken to reduce the risk of kidney damage, such as giving you extra intravenous fluid hydration, and encouraging you to increase the fluids that you drink. This extra fluid helps to quickly flush the medicine out of your system, and ultimately protect your kidneys. Because of the intravenous fluids before and after Cisplatin, the total infusion time might take up to 5 hours.

Cisplatin can also change the taste of certain foods, and may cause a metallic taste in your mouth. Peripheral neuropathy is a side effect of Cisplatin that affects the nervous system and can cause numbness, tingling, burning, pain, or weakness in your hands and/or feet. There are some medications to treat the peripheral neuropathy if it develops. There is a rare chance that Cisplatin can affect hearing and your inner-ear. Let your doctor know immediately if you notice any hearing changes or ringing in the ears.

Cisplatin should be given once in a 21-day cycle (every three weeks), in combination with Pemetrexed. Your doctor will likely want to see you in between treatments. They will look at certain blood values, such as the complete blood count (a simple blood test which calculates the concentration of white blood cells, red blood cells, and platelets in the blood). They might also draw a chemistry panel, which looks at the measures of kidney and liver function and electrolytes (the minerals that help keep the body's fluid levels in balance, and are necessary to help the muscles, heart, and other organs work properly).

Alimta (Pemetrexed)

Pemetrexed is a relatively new chemotherapy. Following years of **clinical trials**, it was approved by the Food and Drug Administration (FDA) in 2004. Pemetrexed can be given alone, but is more commonly given in combination with Cisplatin. It works by interfering with enzymes (proteins that speed up chemical reactions) that the cancer cell needs to replicate. It blocks folate (cancer cells use B-vitamins, such as folate, to make new genetic material), thereby disrupting the cancer cells' ability to grow and replicate. To lower the chances of side effects with Pemetrexed, it is necessary to take folic acid and vitamin B12 before, during, and after treatment. Your doctor will prescribe a folic acid tablet for at least 5 to 7 days before you start Pemetrexed. You will continue taking the folic acid every day until 21 days after your last cycle of Pemetrexed. You will need a B-12 injection within the week before you start the Pemetrexed. B-12 injections will be given about every 9 weeks while you are on this chemotherapy.

Common side effects of Pemetrexed include decreased blood counts, fatigue, as well as nausea and vomiting. Skin reactions, including rash, can also occur, so it's important to let your doctor know if you notice any rash during or after you receive Pemetrexed. Your doctor may prescribe a steroid tablet for you to take the day before, day of, and day after the chemotherapy infusion to lessen the likelihood of skin reactions. Pemetrexed is also associated with decreased appetite and diarrhea. If the diarrhea or vomiting becomes too severe it can cause dehydration (if you lose more fluid

Clinical trial

A type of research study that uses volunteers to test new methods of screening, prevention, diagnosis, or treatment of a disease. The trial may be carried out in a clinic or other medical facility. Also called a clinical study.

than you take in, so your body is so fluid-depleted that it doesn't have enough water to carry out normal function). Mouth sores (stomatitis) can also occur, and you should let your doctor know if they develop, so that they can be treated immediately.

Pemetrexed is given as an intravenous infusion once in a 21-day cycle (every three weeks). The infusion runs over 10 minutes. The dose of the drug will depend on many factors including your age, height, weight, and general health status. Your doctor may see you while you're taking Pemetrexed to examine you and draw a complete blood count, to make sure the drug has not caused your blood cell counts to become too low.

Navelbine is another chemotherapeutic agent which has been shown to have efficacy in mesothelioma. It is usually used after a patient has been given pemetrexed and cisplatin, or if the patient does not have a good performance status. Navelbine is given as an intravenous injection (IV push) or infusion (IV) over 6 to 10 minutes. It is given weekly. There is no oral (by mouth) form. Navelbine is a vesicant (it can cause tissue damage and blistering if it escapes from the vein). If you notice pain, redness or swelling at the IV site during, or after, the Navelbine infusion, alert your doctor immediately. Navelbine can also affect normal cells just like all other chemotherapies, so possible side effects will include low blood counts as well as fatigue, nausea, and hair loss. Navelbine can also cause constipation, so your doctor may prescribe a stool softener or laxative to help with this potential side effect. Joint pain, muscle weakness, or jaw pain can also develop, and should be discussed with your doctor. Like Cisplatin, it can also cause peripheral neuropathy (numbness, tingling, burning, pain, or weakness in your hands and/or feet). Your doctor will likely see you and examine you throughout your treatment with Navelbine, as well as check blood values for side effects of the drug.

The role of radiation in mesothelioma has really been undefined. It has been used to try to control symptoms associated with cancer, such as pain. However, it has not been found to be of benefit as a primary treatment option. Radiation therapy is now being used as part of a combination package with surgery or with surgery and chemotherapy to assess whether it can kill the cancer cells remaining after surgery and prevent the cancer from coming back in the chest. There is much research to be done in this field, and clinical trials are currently underway that are trying to answer these questions and find the best treatment options for people with mesothelioma.

63. What are clinical trials?

Clinical trials are medical research studies that are designed to evaluate new cancer treatments and the effects these treatments have on patients. They are one of the most important ways doctors have to improve care and move forward in the fight against cancer. They are designed to answer specific questions and give information on the safest and most effective ways to treat cancer. Patients who participate in these trials not only make contributions to science but also are able to receive new treatments before they are made available to the general public. The Food and Drug Administration (FDA) oversees these clinical trials and allows certain promising drugs to be used before they are approved for everyday use. All experimental protocols must be thoroughly evaluated by the Investigational Review Board or IRB of the hospital or institution where the study is to be conducted before any patient can be entered into a clinical trial.

A clinical trial has three different steps or phases. The first studies (Phase 1 trials) are the earliest studies of a new treatment. The goal at this stage is to find out the proper dose that should be given and identify potential side effects. The treatment is offered only to patients who have not responded to standard treatments and have widespread disease. Not much is known about the treatment at this stage, and there may be a higher risk of side effects, so these treatments are offered to only a small number of patients.

In a Phase II trial, the new treatment has been found to have some anticancer activity and is being used to treat a particular type of cancer to see how well it works and to obtain more information about its effectiveness and safety. Phase III trials are used to compare the new treatment with the current, standard treatment that has already been proven effective for that type of cancer. In this phase, doctors are trying to find out whether the new treatment is better than or equal to the one that is currently being used. These types of trials have two or more treatments that are being compared, and each treatment becomes one arm of the study. A patient is randomized (assigned by chance, not by choice) to a particular treatment arm or group by the trial; the patient or doctor is not able to influence the assignment.

It is always the patient's decision to enter into a clinical trial. You will never be made part of a trial without your written consent.

64. How do I learn about clinical trials, and how do I decide whether a trial is right for me?

You can learn more about clinical trials by talking with your doctor or by contacting the Cancer Information

Gene therapy
Treatment that alters a gene. In studies of gene therapy for cancer, researchers are trying to improve the body's natural ability to fight the disease or to make the cancer cells more sensitive to other kinds of therapy by either adding a gene which was lost in the cancer or interfering with a gene which contributes to the growth of the cancer.

Service of the National Cancer Institute. This is a free service that is available to you by dialing 1-800-4-CANCER. Many different clinical trials are underway at institutions around the country. You can ask to have a second opinion to talk to other specialists about the trials they are conducting in their area.

Heated chemoperfusion

The delivery of heated chemotherapy chemicals to the chest and/or abdomen in the operating room after the majority of the tumor is removed.

Molecularly targeted therapy

In cancer treatment, substances that kill cancer cells by targeting key molecules involved in cancer cell growth.

Some people associate being in a clinical trial with being used as a "guinea pig" for experimentation. Understanding what is involved with each trial and educating yourself as much as possible before making a decision will help to alleviate some of the fears and anxieties that go along with any clinical trial. Treatment decisions are often difficult to make; therefore it is important to discuss your options with the doctors involved in your care and with family members and others close to you. Although the final decision is yours to make, others may be able to help you think through your options. Write down a list of questions to ask your doctor so you don't forget something during your appointment.

There are certain things you should find out about the trial so that you know what it involves and what is required of you ahead of time. Asking questions may help you decide whether a trial is right for you and may also get rid of some of the uncertainties you may have. Ask the doctor what the specific treatment is and what makes it different from the standard treatments. Also, find out about the specific side effects related to the treatment. You will want to know how long the study will last, whether you have to be hospitalized for the treatment, and where the trial will take place. Lastly, cost is an important consideration for most people. Find out what your insurance will cover before you make your final decision about the trial. The cost of the drugs involved in these trials is usually covered by the study itself, but other expenses may not be covered. You will probably receive more tests and examinations by your doctor when you are in a clinical trial than you would normally receive. This is because your condition and progress must be closely monitored, and study data must be collected at specific intervals along the way. This monitoring is accomplished by following a carefully designed treatment plan called a protocol that spells out what will be done and why.

If you do decide to participate in a clinical trial, you will be given an informed consent form to read over and sign before you are enrolled in the study. The informed consent entails much more than simply obtaining a signature on a form. The key to informed consent is education, as the informed consent serves to reinforce the information given to you by your physician. This document serves to reinforce the information given to you by your physician regarding the trial, including its potential risks and benefits. Signing the consent means that you have received information about the trial and you are freely agreeing to be part of the study. Remember that it is a personal choice to enroll in a study, and therefore you can always refuse to be part of any clinical trial. Also keep in mind that you may withdraw from a study at any time along the way for any reason.

65. What if I don't qualify for a clinical trial?

All clinical trials have 'eligibility criteria' that patients must meet in order to participate. Many factors come into play in determining whether or not a person is eligible for a particular clinical trial. Each protocol has certain specific eligibility criteria. If you don't meet all the criteria, you will not be able to participate in that trial. This means that specific characteristics of your health or your cancer don't match with the study and its requirements. However, this does not necessarily mean that you are ineligible for other clinical trials that are available. If you do not fit into any clinical trial at this time, other treatment options may be available to you that are among the standard treatments for your disease.

66. What are some experimental investigative treatments for mesothelioma?

New agents are being evaluated in mesothelioma, including drugs targeted against certain molecules on the surface of the cells, molecules that help make blood vessels for the tumor, molecules that nourish the tumor, as well as molecules that are involved with immune responses to the tumor. Epidermal growth factor is part of the pathway that helps mesotheliomas grow, and drugs against the molecule that links EGF to the cell (the receptor, EGFr) interfere with this growth pathway. In the majority of cases, there must be a mutation or error in the DNA of the receptor for these drugs to work, and since these errors are not found in mesothelioma, the trials with the EGFr inhibitory drugs have not been encouraging in the disease. Another growth factor associated with platelets, PDGF, has also been the target of a few trials. Vascular endothelial growth factor helps the tumor make blood vessels so it can get more oxygen and nutrients, and there are a number of drugs which are trying to inhibit this characteristic of the tumor. Some of the drugs used for this are small molecules and some are actually proteins called antibodies in order to interfere with either the growth factor or the receptor. There are some characteristic proteins associated with mesothelioma, and using antibodies linked to toxic molecules against these proteins in order to selectively target mesothelioma and not normal tissues. Certain proteins have been found to be uniquely associated with mesothelioma and there are trials in which investigators are attempting to vaccinate patients against these proteins. These vaccination trials attempt to "wakeup" the immune system which is suppressed in mesothelioma and use the immune cells to kill the tumor.

On the surgical side, there are novel therapies also including bathing the chest cavity and the belly with very hot solutions containing chemotherapy in order to try to kill remaining cells. This experimental procedure is under investigation and the results are not in yet.

By the time you read this book there will be other novel molecules that are in the pipeline for mesothelioma. You need to ask you, doctors specifically about novel trials, and then decide yourself if you want to participate in those clinical trials after you hear about the risks and possible benefits.

67. What is alternative therapy?

Alternative and complementary medicines are the use of remedies or therapies that are not considered part of mainstream medicine. They include a broad range of healing philosophies and approaches such as herbal therapy, acupuncture, meditation, and guided imagery. Although both terms are often used interchangeably, there are slight differences in their meaning. Alternative therapy is something that is used in place of or instead of a conventional form of treatment. A complementary therapy is one that is used in addition to rather than in place of a conventional treatment.

Response

The results measured either by x-ray or physical exam of treatment that compares the status (usually the size) of the tumor before treatment to its status after treatment.

68. What should I know about complementary and alternative therapies?

Interest in complementary and alternative therapy has been increasing over the past few years. People diagnosed with many types of diseases, including cancer, are now exploring these options. In the past, there had been very few well-designed studies that looked at the effectiveness and safety of these therapies. What information was available was in the form of anecdotal notes (someone told someone else that the treatment worked). This seems to be changing now as more research is being done in this area. Most patients who decide to use this type of approach will use a complementary therapy in combination with their conventional treatment. Some people choose to use alternative therapies alone as their primary treatment, or to use them after their conventional treatment has failed. Many of these therapies are based on nutrition and diet. The primary goal behind many of these therapies is to try to restore a poorly functioning immune system that is having trouble controlling the growth of the cancer. However, there are conflicting opinions on whether immune system enhancers should be used during active treatment. It is best to talk with your doctor before beginning any type of alternative or complementary therapy. At times, these therapies may interact with the conventional therapy that is prescribed. For example, they may decrease the effectiveness of your treatment or cause more side effects to occur.

69. How do I decide on a treatment plan when faced with multiple options?

Deciding on the best treatment plan for your mesothelioma can be overwhelming, especially when you have been given multiple options. It is in your best interest to take some time to learn about the disease and its treatment. Having a full discussion with your health care team about the extent of your disease, the purpose of treatments, any potential side effects, and the expected results is an important part of the process. The best time to obtain a second opinion is during this stage of decision making, prior to the start of any type of treatment. Your network of family and friends are invaluable during this time and may be able to assist you in making some of these difficult decisions. Ask both your original doctor and the doctors you see for a second opinion about any clinical trials that may be available for you to participate in. Before you decide on a plan of care, you should understand the differences among the treatments and how they compare to one another in terms of possible side effects, risks, benefits, and impact on your current lifestyle. You may use members of your health care team to help you make decisions, but remember: the final choice is yours.

70. How do I know if my treatment is working?

Several different methods are used to determine how well your treatment is working. First, you will be seeing your doctor often during this treatment period and will be having frequent physical exams and lab tests to look for signs of further illness or problems. You will be asked to watch for any unusual or new symptoms and report any of these to your doctor. If some new symptom develops in another site of the body your doctor will order specific tests to evaluate the area.

Before your treatment started, you had x-rays and CT scans performed to learn the extent and size of your disease. The same types of scans will be repeated to analyze these areas and determine whether your cancer has decreased or increased in size or stayed the same during your treatment. In talking about how well the treatment is working, your doctor will speak in terms of the disease's **response** to the treatment. The term "complete response" means that the cancer appears to be completely gone from the body. A "partial response" means that the tumor has shrunk by at least 50% of its original size. With "no response" or stable disease, the cancer has not really grown or shrunk during the treatment. Lastly, if you have "progressive disease," it means that the cancer is growing despite the treatment you have received. By looking at these test results, the doctor gains valuable information about how effective your treatment has been and what the next step should be.

71. What if my disease has remained stable during treatment?

If your disease has remained stable during your treatment—that is, it has not grown or shrunk—the cancer has remained much the same as when you started. Although the ultimate goal of any treatment plan is to rid the body of all of the cancer or as much of it as you can, the fact that your cancer has not continued to grow is a positive sign. The treatment has at least helped to keep the cancer in check and not allowed it to get any worse. If you are in the middle of your treatment, the doctor will probably have you continue on the same therapy until the planned length of treatment is completed. If you are at the end of your current treatment and are being evaluated for the next step in your therapy, a change will be required.

PART SEVEN

Side Effects of Therapy

What can I do about depression, nausea, pain, constipation, and other side effects of therapy?

How should I change my diet following a mesothelioma diagnosis?

What are the benefits of exercise and other activities?

More...

72. Why am I always tired? What can I do for fatigue? Will the fatigue go away after my treatment is over? Could I be depressed?

Fatigue is the one of the most common complaints among cancer patients. People will often say that they can't do the things they used to enjoy doing and that this has affected their lifestyle. There is usually no single cause associated with this fatigue; instead a combination of multiple factors leads to these feelings. These include stress related to the illness and its treatment, symptoms of the disease, nutritional changes, psychological factors such as anxiety and fear, and side effects of treatment. In order to understand cancer fatigue, you must first have an understanding of normal fatigue. This type of fatigue occurs in response to strenuous mental or physical activity and has a protective effect that helps prevent injury. The fatigue seen in people with cancer is much more debilitating. It is an overwhelming sense of exhaustion that does not respond easily to rest and persists over time, causing a decreased ability to perform everyday normal life activities.

It's important to try to find out what is causing your fatigue so that you know what you're dealing with. Fatigue may be the result of the disease itself or its treatment. Mesothelioma can affect your breathing in a number of ways. You may have had lung surgery that has caused you to lose lung tissue, or your disease may be reducing your breathing capacity. This can lead to fatigue because less oxygen is being taken in and less carbon dioxide is going out of the body. Chemotherapy and radiation therapy can also lead to fatigue. Both of these treatments can affect the bone marrow and its ability to make red blood cells. These cells are responsible for carrying oxygen to the tissues in the body. If you have too few red blood cells, the body tissues don't get enough oxygen to do their work, and anemia results. This anemia can cause you to feel weak, tired, short of breath, and dizzy. You may require a blood transfusion to increase the number of red blood cells if your level becomes too low. It's important to let your doctor know if any of these symptoms occur. Your blood counts will be monitored closely while you are receiving your treatment.

Fatigue can also be the result of stress related to your cancer, trips to the hospital for your treatment, uncontrolled pain, and lack of sleep. Here are some strategies you may want to try to combat this problem:

- Limit the activities you do in a day to those that are most important to you.
- Plan uninterrupted rest periods before and after activities to help conserve your energy.
- Get some light exercise, like taking a walk everyday. This will help to increase your energy level. It can also help maintain your muscle tone.
- Talk with others about your fears and concerns, and try to reduce the stresses in your life. You may need to seek professional help for this.
- Make sure you are eating as well as you can. A well-balanced diet that consists of several small meals throughout the day is best. Ask to speak to a dietician if you need help in this area.
- Ask for assistance from your health care team if you are experiencing pain, or sleep difficulties.
- Don't be afraid to ask for help from your family and friends. They can assist you with things like housework, driving, and shopping.

Fatigue caused by the cancer treatment itself usually declines slowly over a period of a few weeks after its completion. Although cancer-related fatigue is often a challenging problem and frustrating to those experiencing it, there are ways to cope with its effects.

Depression is a very common psychological problem that occurs in people with a cancer diagnosis. If you have been feeling depressed for at least two weeks or more, let your doctor know. If you are experiencing mild depression, staying socially active and having a regular exercise routine may help. If your depression is more severe, there are a number of medications that may help. Your doctor may want to start you on one of these medications for a period of time to see if it improves your symptoms. Professional consultation with a counselor may also help you work through your feelings of depression. Remember that you are not alone and that there are many people out there who are able and willing to assist you.

73. Can my shortness of breath be controlled?

Shortness of breath is a common symptom of mesothelioma. A person becomes short of breath when the tissues in his or her body are in need of more oxygen in order to function. This need for oxygen causes a person to start breathing faster and can lead to a feeling of anxiety. This rapid breathing actually makes the problem worse and starts a cycle that can be hard to break. Shortness of breath can be caused by a number of things, including fluid in the space between the lung and chest wall, tumors in the chest itself that encroach on normal lung tissue, anemia, and muscle weakness. There are also other underlying conditions that may cause this problem, such as chronic obstructive pulmonary disease (COPD), emphysema, or heart disease.

Often patients with mesothelioma have one or more of these other medical problems as well that contribute to their overall shortness of breath. It is important to determine the actual cause of the shortness of breath because treatment may be available.

The following are some tips to help you manage your shortness of breath:

- Try using relaxation techniques to relax your muscles, because when your muscles are tense they use more oxygen. Guided imagery, meditation, and the use of relaxation tapes are good examples.
- Take frequent rests when you are walking or performing any physical exercise.
- Sleep on more than one pillow so that your head is raised above your shoulders.
- Let your doctor know if you are experiencing shortness of breath, as he or she may suggest oxygen or medications to help ease your breathing.
- Practice controlled breathing to help you feel as though you are getting enough air. Start with a normal breath and count the seconds it takes you to inhale through your nose. Then exhale normally through pursed lips for twice as long as you inhaled.

74. What can I do to relieve my pain?

Patients with mesothelioma can have tumors that are invasive. These tumors will actually grow into muscles and nerves and can cause pain by doing so. There have been many advances over the years that have helped ensure that patients with pain get adequate relief. Today, many options are available to help manage pain.

Although not all cancer patients experience serious problems with pain, there are those that do. Cancer pain may occur suddenly (acute pain) or continuously over a period of time (chronic pain). It can have a variety of causes, such as the cancer itself, the treatment, or an underlying condition such as arthritis.

Pain is a very individual thing, and no two people experience it in exactly the same way. A lot of unique variables come into play and affect how you feel. Some of these include the physical cause of the pain, your culture and its attitudes toward pain, and your previous experiences and understanding of pain and its treatment. How other people respond to you and support you when you are having pain also affects how you feel. Pain can prevent you from sleeping, eating, and enjoying time with your friends and family.

You can play an important role in controlling your pain by expressing your feelings and describing the pain to your health care team. Remember that treating pain right away is more effective than waiting until it becomes severe. Be as specific as possible so that the best method of pain control for your type of pain is utilized. Tell your doctor where the pain is located; the type of pain you're having, such as dull, sharp, or burning; how often it occurs; how long it lasts; and anything that aggravates or relieves it. Pain may feel worse when you are tired, anxious, worried, or depressed. Talking through your emotions with those close to you may help. Also, you may find some relief after using relaxation techniques. If your pain is not helped by lighter pain medications such as Tylenol or Advil, your doctor may start you on prescription medicines. Many different types of medications, such as narcotics, antidepressants, and anticonvulsants, are used to treat pain.

They are available in many different forms, such as orally (by mouth), as patches placed on the skin, as suppositories (medication given via the rectum), or by injection. These medicines, like many others, also have side effects. The most common side effects seen in people who are taking narcotic pain medication are constipation, nausea and vomiting, and sleepiness.

Pain can also change over time, and controlling it can require a number of different treatment plans. Many hospitals have pain teams or clinics that specialize in the treatment of pain, and your doctor may send you to see these professionals. Sometimes pain can't be controlled with medications, and other treatments such as nerve blocks (to block pain due to nerve compression), surgery, or radiation (used to shrink the tumor) can be used. The main goal of any pain regimen is to control pain with the maximum amount of relief and a minimum of side effects. Your doctor will work with you to find the most effective treatment for your individual pain needs.

75. What can I do to prevent or relieve constipation?

Constipation is a common side effect that occurs in people who are taking narcotic pain medications or who are receiving chemotherapy treatment for their cancer. Contributing to the problem is the fact that you may be less active and not eating as well as you normally would. It is important to drink plenty of fluids and stick to high-fiber foods such as fruits and vegetables, nuts, and whole-wheat breads and cereals. Try to avoid foods that can cause constipation, such as cheese. Don't forget about those old-time remedies, such as prunes or prune juice and bran. If possible, exercise by simply getting outside and taking a walk. You may need to take stool softeners and laxatives on a daily basis, especially if you are taking narcotic pain medications. Be sure to take these as recommended and not just when you feel you need them. In some cases, if these remedies are not effective, you may require an enema or suppository. Let your doctor know if you haven't had a bowel movement in three or more days, and check with him or her before taking any of these remedies.

76. Am I at risk for a blood clot? What is a pulmonary embolism?

People diagnosed with mesothelioma may be more prone to developing blood clots. This is because they can have more platelets (cells that cause the blood to clot) in their bloodstream than normal. Also, they may be more debilitated and may not be getting up and moving around enough. Often, blood clots form in the legs and cause the legs and feet to swell. Blood clots can be very serious, and once they occur they have the ability to move through the bloodstream to other organs, such as the lungs, heart, or rarely brain. If a clot breaks off and travels to the lung it can cause a pulmonary embolism. This is a blockage of the lung artery or one of its branches caused by a blood clot. A pulmonary embolism can be fatal, so it's very important to identify and treat blood clots as soon as possible. Blood clots can be treated with medications that cause the blood to become thin and therefore reduce the chance of a clot developing. Heparin is the drug that is used initially, followed by Coumadin. While on Coumadin, you will require frequent blood tests to make sure you are receiving the right amount of the drug. Because of this risk of blood clots, make sure to report any symptoms of swelling in the legs and feet or any sudden onset of shortness of breath to your doctor immediately.

77. Will I have terrible nausea and vomiting during my chemotherapy treatment?

For many years chemotherapy has been automatically associated with nausea and vomiting. Although these side effects are common, not all chemotherapy drugs cause nausea and vomiting, and not every person will experience these symptoms. It is true that these drugs are very powerful, and many of them can cause nausea, episodes of vomiting, or both. However, there are a number of new medications on the market today that control nausea and vomiting much more effectively than their older counterparts did. Preventing nausea and vomiting is much easier than trying to get it under control once it happens. Therefore, before you even start your chemotherapy treatment, you will be given antinausea medications to help prevent you from getting sick. Chemotherapy can affect the stomach, the vomiting control center in the brain, or both. A wide variety of drugs is available to control or lessen these effects. Not all drugs work the same for all people, and it may be necessary to change the drug you are on or use more than one in combination to get relief. Some people experience slight nausea most of the time, while others become severely nauseated for a limited time after the chemotherapy dose. Symptoms may start soon after treatment or 8 to 12 hours later and may last only a few hours or up to 24 hours after the therapy is given. Some people may even start to feel sick before their treatment starts. This is called **anticipatory nausea**. It is important to let your doctor or nurse know if you are experiencing severe nausea or have vomited for more than a day. If you are unable to keep liquids down, you may become dehydrated and need to have

Anticipatory nausea and vomiting (ANV)

ANV is nausea and/or vomiting that occur prior to the beginning of a new cycle of chemotherapy, in response to conditioned stimuli such as the smells, sights, and sounds of the treatment room. ANV is a classically conditioned response that typically occurs after 3 or 4 prior chemotherapy treatments, following which the person experienced acute or delayed N&V.

fluids given to you intravenously. Severe dehydration may even require you to be hospitalized. Here are some suggestions for ways to limit your symptoms:

- Try eating small, frequent meals throughout the day so your stomach doesn't feel too full.
- Eat your meals slowly and drink fluids at least an hour before or after your meals instead of with them.
- Avoid strong odors such as perfume or cooking smells.
- Wear clothing that is loose and doesn't bind.
- Distract yourself by using relaxation techniques or by watching television or listening to music.
- Eat foods cold or at room temperature and avoid fried, sweet, or fatty foods or those that are strong tasting.
- If you are nauseated, try eating mild foods, such as crackers or toast.

Talk with your health care provider and work with him or her to find the treatment that is best for you.

78. Will I lose my hair during chemotherapy or radiation?

Hair loss is another common side effect of cancer treatment and can be one of the most traumatic. Although it's not harmful to the body, it is a constant visual reminder of the effects of cancer and its treatment and can significantly alter the way you look. Your doctor can tell you whether the chemotherapy drugs you are to receive are likely to cause hair loss. Alopecia (hair loss) occurs because chemotherapy causes the hair follicles to weaken, and thus hair falls out more quickly than normal. Since hair follicles have rapidly dividing cells, they may be damaged during chemotherapy resulting in hair loss. If hair loss does occur, certain areas such as the head or the entire body may be affected, including the eyelashes and eyebrows. The hair can become thinner or it can be lost completely. Hair loss will usually begin anywhere from one week to several weeks after treatment and may occur gradually or in clumps.

Hair loss associated with chemotherapy is usually temporary. Your hair will start to grow back after your treatments are over, but it may take four to six months to do so. Sometimes it may even start to grow back while you are still receiving your chemotherapy. The new hair may be a different texture, color, or thickness when it grows back, but these changes are not usually permanent.

Radiation therapy can also cause hair thinning or loss of hair, but it does not occur over the entire body. Only the area that is directly under the radiation beam will be affected. Therefore, if you are receiving radiation to the chest the hair loss will occur in the chest area. The hair on your head will be affected only if you are receiving radiation to the head or scalp. Hair may start to fall out two to three weeks after the radiation starts. Usually it will start to grow back after radiation treatments are completed, but if the dose of radiation you received was high the hair loss may be permanent.

Before treatment begins, you may want to look into buying a wig or hairpiece. This is the best time to see a professional hairdresser or wig consultant because he or she will be able to match the color and style to your real hair. The American Cancer Society has wigs that they loan to people, so if this interests you, give them a call.

Side Effects of Therapy

It might be helpful to have your hair cut shorter to make hair loss easier to manage if it should happen. Some people try wearing bandanas, scarves, or hats. These are all ways to help you feel normal during your cancer treatment. Do what feels most comfortable for you. During your chemotherapy, try to use mild shampoos, soft hairbrushes, and low heat when using a hair dryer, and avoid the use of hair dye. Losing your hair can be difficult and can cause you to feel angry or depressed. Talking about your feelings with those you trust may help.

79. Is my cough something I should worry about?

A cough is one of the symptoms that can occur with mesothelioma, and it can result from fluid pressing on the lung or from the tumor mass irritating the pleura. A change in the pattern of an existing cough may be an important warning sign and should be followed up on. During the course of your illness, the underlying reason for your cough may change. This is why it is necessary to let your doctor know about any differences as soon as they happen. In order to treat your cough as effectively as possible, it is important to identify the cause.

As we noted previously, your cough may be caused by fluid that is around your lung in the pleural space. If your doctor performs a procedure to remove this fluid, your cough may improve or disappear. However, if your cough returns or becomes worse, this may be one of the first signs that the fluid has come back. Your doctor may order a chest x-ray to evaluate the situation and may perform another procedure to try to get rid of the fluid. When no specific, treatable cause for the cough is found, the doctor may prescribe a cough suppressant.

80. What can I do if I have lost my appetite?

Mesothelioma and its treatment can cause a loss of normal appetite (**anorexia**). There are a number of specific reasons why you may lose your appetite. These include tumor growth, depression, difficulty swallowing, pain, nausea, and changes in taste and smell. Chemotherapy can cause the normal cells that line your mouth, stomach, and intestines to be altered or destroyed. This may, in turn, cause the food and fluids that you take in to taste different. They may take on a metallic or bitter taste or may seem very sweet. You may also lose your desire to eat, but this is usually temporary and improves over a period of two to six weeks after your chemotherapy is finished.

It is very important for you to eat as much as you can in order to maintain your weight. Those who eat well seem to be able to cope better and fight off infection easier. If you find something that tastes good and you can eat it without difficulty, then do so. Eat anything you want and as much as you want. The following is a list of suggestions to help you manage your loss of appetite:

- Snack frequently throughout the day, and eat whenever you feel like you can.
- Eat high-calorie and high-protein foods and snacks, such as nuts, eggs, cheese, peanut butter, and milkshakes. Try adding protein powders to your drinks.
- Add butter or margarine, creams, and gravies to your meals to boost calories.
- Let other people fix your meals so you are able to conserve your energy and stay away from cooking odors.
- Do some light exercise, like walking, about an hour before you eat, to stimulate your appetite.

Anorexia

An abnormal loss of the appetite for food. Anorexia can be caused by cancer, AIDS, a mental disorder (i.e., anorexia nervosa), or other diseases.

Side Effects of Therapy

- Drink plenty of fluids, but try to drink them between meals instead of with them because they can contribute to your feelings of fullness.
- Use plastic utensils instead of metal if your food tastes metallic.
- Eat with friends or family whenever possible, as socializing helps to increase appetite. When you are eating alone, watch TV or have the radio on.
- Vary your mealtime routine and try new foods and recipes.
- Use food supplements like Ensure if you are able to. They are high in calories and nutrients.

**Cachexia
(ka-KEK-see-a)**

Loss of body weight and muscle mass, and weakness that may occur in patients with cancer, AIDS, or other chronic diseases. Cachexia is a common manifestation of late stage mesothelioma.

Anorexia can lead to a very serious problem for people with cancer called **cachexia** (a condition that causes a breakdown in muscle mass in those with chronic illness). Weight loss is a symptom of cancer and a side effect of treatment, but if left unchecked it can lead to cachexia. Your doctor may have to start you on a medication, like Megace, to help stimulate your appetite. Be sure to discuss any appetite problems with your doctor, and notify him or her if you are losing weight.

81. Are there long-term side effects from treatment?

Most side effects that are experienced as a result of surgery resolve in a few days to a few weeks after the operation. Pain, however, is one side effect that may last for longer periods of time. Pain at the incision site is an expected outcome of chest surgery, but some people complain of lasting pain that is sometimes harder to eliminate. You will be provided with effective pain medication that you will continue to take at home when you are discharged. Your doctor will work with you to find the most effective medications to help relieve any discomfort that you may have.

Chemotherapy and radiation work to destroy cancer cells but also damage normal cells at the same time. Fortunately, normal cells recover quickly and side effects gradually disappear after treatment ends. The length of time it takes to feel better and regain your energy will vary. Many times side effects go away very quickly, but certain ones may take months or years to recede completely. Other times the treatment may cause side effects that result in permanent damage and can last a lifetime. Sometimes chemotherapy can cause permanent damage to the lungs, kidneys, or heart, depending on the type of chemotherapy you receive and your body's response to it. A specific side effect of chemotherapy, peripheral neuropathy, may cause difficulty with balance or gain and can also make it difficult to pick up and handle objects. If you develop peripheral neuropathy, the symptoms may improve after the completion of chemotherapy, but they might not totally go away.

It is important to keep in mind that many people don't experience any long-term problems. The unwanted effects of treatment may not be pleasant, but they must be compared to the benefits of treatment and its ability to destroy the cancer. Talk with your doctor or nurse if you have any questions about side effects or the way you are feeling after treatment.

82. How should I change my diet following a mesothelioma diagnosis? Should I take dietary supplements? Can diet affect my survival?

Eating well, although it can be challenging at times, enables you to cope better with the disease and its treatment. It is important that you drink a lot of fluids and eat as much as you can so that you are able to maintain your weight and keep your strength up. This means that you should pick a variety of foods that contain protein, calories, vitamins, and minerals to keep your body functioning properly. Protein-enriched foods help build and repair body tissues that are injured. If your calorie intake is too low, the body uses protein for energy first, and there may not be enough left to repair the tissues.

Cancer is known to affect a person's metabolism, even though the mechanism for this is not clear. Some nutrition experts say that during treatment a person may require up to 50% more protein and 20% more calories than normal. It has been shown that patients who are able to eat and drink well are better able to handle the side effects of treatment and can fight off infection more easily by strengthening the immune system. Also, it can make a big difference in a person's outlook and quality of life.

Nutritional supplements may help fill the gap in nutrients that are missing from your diet. This gap may be due to a lack of appetite or depletion of key nutrients because of stress or certain medications you are on. Some people may benefit from taking vitamin and mineral supplements, but before doing so you should check with your doctor. High doses of certain vitamins and minerals can be toxic or can react with treatment medications. Ask to speak to a dietician if you have specific nutritional questions or need assistance with your diet.

83. What are the benefits of exercise for mesothelioma patients?

Exercise is an important consideration for all people, whether they are currently healthy and disease free or are diagnosed with cancer and undergoing treatment.

You may already have a regular exercise routine that you follow, and if you have surgery, your doctors should encourage you to get back into an exercise routine. If you are able to continue with your previous routine, then do so; however, you may find it necessary to adjust it somewhat. Keep in mind that any type of light exercise is useful and may help to decrease your feelings of fatigue and stimulate your appetite. Walking is an exercise that is usually well tolerated, and you should walk as much as possible. One way you can give your arms some exercise is by lifting light weights. If the muscles in your chest and arms are sore, you can also use exercises such as slow stretching or walking your fingers up a wall to relieve this. It is important to talk with your doctor before starting on any exercise program.

84. What about returning to work?

Work is an important part of life for many people and can provide a sense of purpose and financial security. Also, many psychological and social needs are met at the workplace.

Some people who are diagnosed with mesothelioma are able to return to work at some point, either during or after treatment. Your doctor may place restrictions on the activities or job duties that you can perform based on limitations you may have. When returning to work, you may also be faced with issues such as how to talk about your disease and its treatment with coworkers and how to deal with their reactions. It might be helpful for you to plan ahead and work through some of these concerns beforehand. Discuss your individual needs and work situation with your doctor. He or she will let you know if and when you can return to work and will help in any way possible.

85. What about follow-up care? How often should I be seen?

All patients with mesothelioma who receive treatment should be monitored very closely during and after treatment, whether they participate in a clinical trial or not. If you are on a specific clinical trial, the follow-up schedule will be clearly defined in the protocol and will be explained to you before you start the trial. During treatment with chemotherapy, most patients will have weekly blood levels drawn and will be seen by the doctor every two to three weeks. You will receive a physical exam and blood work when you come to see the doctor and will be asked to report any new symptoms you may be having.

A CT scan will usually be performed after two cycles of chemotherapy to see how the cancer is responding to the treatment. If your cancer appears to be getting worse, the doctor will stop the chemotherapy that you are receiving and develop a new plan. If you complete all the treatment you were to receive, the doctor will perform another CT scan and will again evaluate the tumor's response to the treatment. When your therapy has been completed, you will still be monitored with CT scans at regular intervals, along with follow-up visits with your doctor.

In between visits, you need to notify your doctor of any new problems you may be experiencing as soon as they develop. Depending on the symptom you are having, your doctor may order a CT scan earlier than you normally would have one, to evaluate you for any possible cancer growth. If your cancer returns or becomes worse, you may have to receive more treatment. Your doctor will discuss your options with you at that time.

86. Should I get a flu shot or pneumonia vaccine?

Yearly flu shots are recommended for anyone who is 50 years of age or older or has a chronic illness and whose immune system may be compromised. People with a diagnosis of cancer fall into this category and are encouraged to ask their doctor for a flu shot every year. If you have never received the pneumonia vaccine in the past, it is a good idea to receive this vaccine as well. If you have received the pneumonia vaccine before, you will be asked how long ago you received it. If it has been five years or more you should be vaccinated again. It is currently recommended that a person receive only two lifetime doses of the vaccine, so if you have had it twice already, you do not need it repeated.

PART EIGHT

Recurrence of the Disease

What happens if my disease recurs?

Where is my disease likely to recur?

How is recurrence treated?

More . . .

87. What happens if my disease recurs?

With every cancer diagnosis comes the fear that the cancer treatment won't work or that the cancer will eventually return. When people are faced with the diagnosis of recurrent cancer, they experience some of the same emotions that were seen with the original diagnosis, like anger and shock, all over again. These are normal reactions that occur when a person is faced with such a difficult challenge. The difference for you now is that you have been through a similar experience before and have dealt with cancer and the life-altering effects it can have. Obtaining knowledge about the disease and its treatments may help to control some of the emotional and physical reactions you may have. Medical and emotional support is available to you, so try to utilize those around you as much as you can.

When cancer recurs, it becomes active again in the body after a period of inactivity or dormancy. This can happen quickly over weeks or months, or it can take longer and occur years later. Recurrent cancers begin with abnormal cells that start to grow and multiply quickly, much like the original cancer. These recurrent tumors start from cells that originated from the first cancer. These cells were either left behind after treatment was completed, either because they were too small to see or because they broke away from the primary tumor and traveled through the lymphatic system or bloodstream to other parts of the body.

Local recurrence

Reappearance of the previously treated cancer at its original site; with mesothelioma, a local recurrence occurs in the pleura most frequently after surgery for the tumor.

Recurrent cancers are classified by location because not only do they differ in their ability to recur but they also differ in the place where they are likely to recur. If the cancer has returned to the same area of the body that it started in, it is called a **local recurrence**. It also means that it is isolated to that area and has not spread to other tissues. A cancer that involves new growth in nearby lymph nodes or tissues near the original site of the cancer is called a **regional recurrence**. Lastly, if the cancer is now found in other organs or tissues that are at some distance from the original site, it is called a **metastatic recurrence**. The treatment you receive now will depend on many factors, including where the disease has recurred, what treatments are available, and your overall health status.

88. Where is my disease likely to recur?

Mesothelioma is a disease that likes to come back to the same area that it originated in. Therefore, if it was first diagnosed in your chest cavity, that is where it will most likely return. The other problem with the disease is that it likes to grow in old wound sites. This process is known as **malignant seeding** and is a common complication of procedures performed on patients with mesothelioma. The areas that your doctor needs to monitor for any signs of possible recurrence include thoracentesis tracts, biopsy tracts, chest tube sites, and surgical incisions. This is why your doctor will ask to feel and look at these sites during your physical exam. Also, be sure to alert your doctor to any new or abnormal lumps or bumps that you notice in these areas. Spread to distant metastatic sites can occur, but this usually happens late in the course of the disease.

After treatment in the chest, the disease can start to grow in the belly. Difficulty in closing skirts or pants at the waist, loss of appetite, and a feeling of fullness can be the harbinger that fluid is building up in the abdomen and that the disease has spread there.

It is important that you follow up with your doctor and are monitored on a regular basis. You should be

Regional recurrence

Return of the cancer in a location close to the original cancer.

Metastatic recurrence

Return of the cancer at a site away from the original site.

Malignant seeding

Growth of a tumor at a site which may be outside its original domain because of contamination of a new site with malignant cells after a biopsy or from cells in a malignant effusion.

having CT scans performed regularly after your treatment in order to evaluate your progress and to check for any possible recurrence.

89. How is recurrence treated?

If your disease recurs, your doctor will discuss what treatments are now available for you. The treatment options will depend upon the size and location of your cancer, what treatments you have already received, and your overall health status. The types of treatments that are recommended to you may include surgery, chemotherapy, or radiation therapy. You should discuss the options thoroughly with your doctor, including what the goals of treatment are and what the possible effects may be.

Surgery is usually reserved for those people who have recurrences at previous incision sites. It may be possible for your surgeon to remove these local recurrences as long as there is no evidence of spread to any other areas. Sometimes surgery is followed by radiation therapy to that area to try to kill cells that may have been left behind.

Many times, doctors are able to treat the recurrent cancer with different forms of the same therapy, such as different chemotherapy drugs than you had the first time. If the cancer is causing symptoms such as pain, then treatment, such as radiation, of these specific areas may be recommended.

Ask your doctor to tell you about any clinical trials that may be available, as new studies may have opened since your original diagnosis. Many people who have faced these decisions a second time have said that knowledge and understanding were again key factors in assisting them through the process. Find out all you can about your cancer and the options you have, so you can make informed decisions and meet this challenge again.

PART NINE

Sue Vento's Insights for Care Providers

Where do I turn for support in dealing with
my own stress and anxiety?

How do I balance all of the responsibilities?

What specific thing can family
and friends do to assist?

More . . .

90. Where do I turn for support in dealing with my own stress and anxiety?

If you are employed, check to see if an Employee Assistance Program (EAP) is available through your employer or your insurance plan. Religious professionals, family therapists and psychologists, and hospice and health organizations such as the American Cancer Society are also possible sources of counseling and assistance.

91. Knowing that this will be an especially stressful time for everyone in the family, what can I do to keep us connected and close?

Small family dinners—preferably potluck and no fuss—as well as other quiet times visiting or playing cards or board games will be comforting. Keep such gatherings brief and flexible, and base them on the patient's desire to have company.

A number of family events occurred during Bruce's treatments. Family members and friends were great in recognizing that our participation depended on how he felt. Everyone was most patient with last-minute changes in plans.

92. What about those inevitable middle-of-the-night situations when my loved one is in pain or has other medical complications?

Do not hesitate to contact your doctor or medical facility at any hour of the day. Such contacts are expected and will be handled promptly. It's helpful to have the names and phone numbers—daytime, nighttime, and weekend—for the doctors, medical facilities, and pharmacies you are dealing with. Knowing which pharmacies are open 24 hours is good information to have before you need it.

I recall several middle-of-the-night phone conversations with Mayo Clinic doctors, as well as a couple of trips to the local 24-hour Walgreen's.

93. How do we focus on the positive while preparing for the worst?

This is a difficult question for which there are no absolute or easy answers. Each individual deals uniquely with the reality of serious illness and death. That's true for the patient as well as his or her family members and friends. However, the patient needs to know who she or he can turn to discuss concerns and requests regarding the diagnosis, the treatment options, the living will, and the painful issues related to death. Religious and hospice professionals can be wonderful sources of wise and healing insight into dealing with these issues.

Early one morning, about a week prior to Bruce's surgery, as we were driving to Rochester for some pre-surgery tests at the Mayo Clinic, we discussed what type of funeral arrangements Bruce wanted. It wasn't as difficult a discussion as you might imagine, and to a great extent, it was a relief for both of us to have faced that subject early in this uncertain journey.

94. How do I balance all of the responsibilities?

Don't even begin to think of doing it all yourself. Allow supportive family and friends to assist. If they offer, say, "Yes, please!" And when in need, ask for assistance.

I quickly quit apologizing for a less than pristine house and for not having coffee or food to serve when visitors came. Those who did visit were not there for inspections or sustenance of any kind! Family and friends recognize that you have more than enough to keep you busy.

Recently I read in a local newspaper about a wonderful foundation called Cleaning for a Reason, which is available to many cancer patients throughout the country. They provide cleaning assistance—as they describe it, "one less thing to worry about." For more information, go to their website at **http://cleaningforareason.org**. If your community is not on their list, it may be possible to change that with a few phone calls! This foundation also accepts contributions.

95. What else can I do to make my loved one comfortable?

I carried a chair cushion to church and gatherings. Bruce lost a significant amount of weight during the chemotherapy and radiation therapy and found sitting to be quite uncomfortable. Carrying along a sweater or jacket as well as medications was important. Because all of the appointments except Bruce's radiation therapy were a significant distance from home, we found it de-stressing to bring an overnight bag for each of us. On a couple of occasions there was fluid buildup or some other condition that made it necessary for Bruce to stay in the hospital.

96. How can family and friends help without intruding?

Ask what might help. Let the patient and his or her care provider know that you want them to be direct with you about what's helpful and what isn't. Call ahead before visiting at home or at the hospital. Keep visits brief and upbeat. When you sense that your loved one is tiring or needing to tend to personal care, depart.

Avoid emotional issues or difficult conversations that will add to the patient's stress and anxiety. If a sensitive conversation needs to occur, talk with the care provider first to determine when and how best to approach it.

97. What specific things can family and friends do to assist?

Staying with the patient while his or her spouse or care provider takes a break, returns to work, runs errands, or attends church or temple will be deeply appreciated. Some families develop a schedule for this as well as a schedule for bringing meals to the patient and family at home. When bringing food, please keep in mind that many times the patient's food preferences will change drastically as a result of chemotherapy, radiation and medications. Bruce found seasoned and spicy foods that he had previously loved became very hard to eat and digest. The "comfort foods" became standard fair.

Day-to-day tasks around the house and yard—laundry, lawn and/or garden care, snow or leaf removal, grocery shopping, and house keeping—are also possible ways to provide much-needed assistance. Providing rides and assistance to and from medical appointments may also be appreciated.

PART TEN

The Unspeakable Which Must Be Spoken

How do I decide when it's time to stop treatment?

What is hospice?

Where can I go to get more information?

More . . .

98. How do I decide when it's time to stop treatment?

Mesothelioma is a disease that can be difficult to control. Treatments may work for a period of time and slow the growth of the cancer, but at some point the disease may come back or become worse. Your doctor may have told you that your cancer can no longer be controlled or that they are no longer able to get ahead of the cancer because of its growth pattern. If this is the situation, you and your doctor may need to think about switching the focus of care to the control of your symptoms and make the decision to stop any other types of aggressive therapy. If your disease and its treatment are causing a significant amount of symptoms that are decreasing your quality of life, you may also choose not to take any further treatment. It can be very difficult to make these types of decisions and have to focus on end-of-life care, but it can also give a person a sense of peace and freedom. This is a good time to do those things you've wanted to do but have been putting off to deal with at a later date. You and your family can make decisions about the future and get your financial and legal affairs in order. This is a good time to talk with your doctor about the types of assistance or programs that are available to you and your family to help take care of your health care needs.

99. What is hospice?

The goal of hospice care is to provide comfort to patients and their families. Hospice is able to provide support and guidance and ensure that all physical, emotional, and spiritual needs are addressed. The treatment focus now switches from control or cure of the disease to palliation or relief of symptoms and quality of life. If you decide that you do not want any more active treatment for your cancer, or if your doctor tells you that your cancer can no longer be controlled, it may be time to consider hospice. A large number of hospice programs exist throughout the country, and even smaller communities usually have hospice care available. To be eligible for hospice, your doctor must state that you are at the end stages of your cancer and have less than six months to live. This is a guideline they use because it is difficult to give an actual estimate of the amount of time a person has before death. To receive the best total care that hospice can provide a patient, it is best to utilize their services months before a person dies rather than in the last few weeks or days. Ask your doctor about hospice care and what is available in your area. The American Cancer Society is also a good resource and can give you information on hospice services.

Sue adds . . .

I was totally clueless when I heard Bruce's doctor at the Mayo Clinic advise us that it was time to get hospice care. When the fog cleared, I was relieved to find the many resources available to us through hospice.

Hospice services frequently include equipment that can be used in the home (beds, walkers, oxygen machines and supplies, and so on), daily or weekly visits by health care aides, nurses, and clergy and counseling staff, and assistance with routine daily hygiene and medical procedures. You or your loved ones may find it advantageous to explore the hospice options in your area well in advance of any need for hospice services. Having to make such contacts, complete the paperwork, and so forth, can be a bit overwhelming once the time comes.

The health aide who visited our homes several mornings a week was a godsend! She assisted Bruce with his shower, shaving, and medical procedures while I caught up on laundry and other errands. The hospice nurse provided helpful suggestions for food alternatives when the nausea increased, options for dealing with constipation and other digestive problems, and advice on the amount and timing of pain medication.

100. The battle is just beginning. Where can I go to get more information?

The next section lists some recommended resources for finding out more about mesothelioma.

Recommended resources for learning more about mesothelioma

Books

An Air That Kills: How the Asbestos Poisoning of Libby, Montana Uncovered a National Scandal, by Andrew Schneider and David McCumber (New York: G. P. Putnam's Sons, 2004).

Outrageous Misconduct: The Asbestos Industry on Trial, by Paul Brodeur (New York: Knopf, 1985).

Dust to Dust, DVD, by Michael Brown (Arlington, TX: Michael Brown Productions, 2002).

Organizations

The Mesothelioma Applied Research Foundation (Meso Foundation), is the national nonprofit organization whose mission is "to eradicate mesothelioma as a life-ending disease." Meso Foundation funds medical research grants to physicians and scientists working to find treatment options and ultimately a cure for this disease. Meso Foundation also provides information, encouragement, and support to patients and family members, and works to increase awareness of and federal research funding for mesothelioma. For more information about Meso Foundation, go to www.curemeso.org or call 805.563.8400.

Cleaning for a Reason is a nonprofit foundation dedicated to providing assistance with house cleaning for cancer patients who need "one less thing to worry about." Based in Texas, this organization has a nationwide network of individuals and companies who volunteer their cleaning services. For more information, call 1-877-337-3348 or go to http://cleaningforareason.org.

http://www.cancer.gov/search

Internet Resources

www.cancer.gov/cancertopics/types/malignantmesothelioma
www.cancer.gov/search/ResultsClinicalTrials.aspx?
protocolsearchid=5639470—For the latest in clinical trials which are sponsored by the National Cancer Institute of the National Institutes of Health, you should use the above websites. The first one will take you to the mesothelioma homesite for the NCI and the second will take you right to the mesothelioma trials.

www.ewg.org—The Environmental Working Group's web site has extensive information about the presence of asbestos in this country as well as information regarding legislative efforts, etc.

www.asbestostruth.net—This web site provides a myriad of info and resources regarding asbestos, mesothelioma, asbestosis, and asbestos cancer as well as doctors, clinical trials, legal resources and state resources.

www.curemeso.org—The web site for the Mesothelioma Applied Research Foundation.

www.CaringBridge.org—CaringBridge is a free Internet service that helps families and friends keep in touch with loved ones battling serious illnesses. In addition to the updates, it includes a guest book where family and friends can return messages of support.

Quotes

"Into my heart an air that kills from yon far country blows."

—A. E. Housman, A Shropshire Lad

"When you think you can't breathe, nothing else matters."

—The American Lung Association

"Pray for the dead and fight like hell for the living."

—Mother Jones

"Our family is a circle of strength and love. With every birth and every union, the circle grows. Every joy shared adds more love. Every crisis faced together makes the circle stronger."

—Unknown

Appendix A: The Information Card

Patient's Name
Address
Daytime & Evening Phone Numbers

Health Insurance Company
Health Insurance Number

Immediate Next-of-Kin/Contact
Daytime & Evening & Cell Phone Numbers

Allergies

Current Medications

Oncologist & Phone Numbers

Surgeon & Phone Numbers

Other Physicians & Health Care Professionals & Phone Numbers

Medical Facility(ies)

Attorney & Phone Numbers

Pharmacy—Names & Phone Numbers

Family members/neighbors/friends/work colleagues:
- Name   Phone number(s)
- Name   Phone number(s)
- Name   Phone number(s)
- Name   Phone number(s)
- Name   Phone number(s)
- Name   Phone number(s)

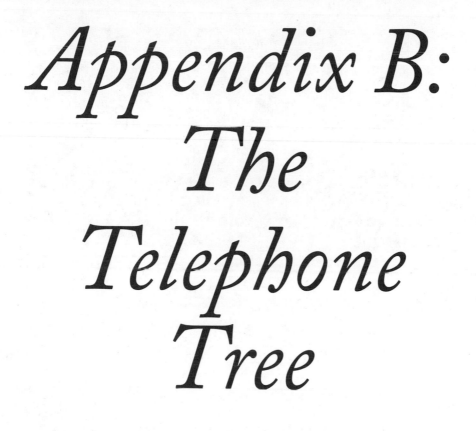

Appendix B: The Telephone Tree

Mesothelioma patients are deluged with a tremendous amount of information and it becomes overwhelming to relate and repeat this to loved ones. We had Bruce's family—his 3 sons, his parents and seven sibling plus my mother and five siblings. The phone calls were initially more exhausting than all the appointments. We quickly figured out that we needed a "phone tree!" It saved us time and energy and the difficulty of repeated conversations after an already exhausting day and it also gave others an opportunity to assist and stay informed.

I suggest that the patient not be in the phone tree. If s/he chooses to start the tree, fine, but in anticipation of the reality that s/he may not be up to it, I suggest that the spouse or care provider be the one to initiate the phone tree communication.

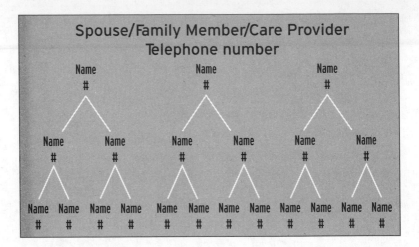

Glossary

Copyright and Registered Trademarks Most of the information on the National Cancer Institute's (NCI's) Web site has been written by federal government employees. This material is in the public domain and is not subject to copyright restrictions. Therefore, no special permission is required to use it or reproduce it. However, any reproduced material should contain proper acknowledgement of NCI as the originator and the NCI Web site, www.cancer.gov, as the source.

A

Adjuvant therapy (AD-joo-vant): Treatment given after the primary treatment to increase the chances of a cure. Adjuvant therapy may include chemotherapy, radiation therapy, hormone therapy, or biological therapy.

Alternative medicine: Practices used instead of standard treatments which are generally not recognized by the medical community as standard or conventional medical approaches. Alternative medicine includes dietary supplements, megadose vitamins, herbal preparations, special teas, acupuncture, massage therapy, magnet therapy, spiritual healing, and meditation.

Anemia (a-NEE-mee-a): A condition in which the number of red blood cells is below normal.

Anorexia: An abnormal loss of the appetite for food. Anorexia can be caused by cancer, AIDS, a mental disorder (i.e., anorexia nervosa), or other diseases.

Anticipatory nausea and vomiting (ANV): ANV is nausea and/or vomiting that occur prior to the beginning of a new cycle of chemotherapy, in response to conditioned stimuli such as the smells, sights, and sounds of the treatment room. ANV is a classically conditioned response that typically occurs after 3 or 4 prior chemotherapy treatments, following which the person experienced acute or delayed N&V.

Arrhythmia: An arrhythmia is any deviation from or disturbance of the normal heart rhythm.

Ascites (ah-SYE-teez): Abnormal build-up of fluid in the abdomen that may cause swelling. In late-stage cancer, tumor cells may be found in the fluid in the abdomen. Ascites is a common manifestation of peritoneal mesothelioma and can occur as a manifestation of recurrent mesothelioma after surgery for the disease in the chest.

B

Biomarker: A substance sometimes found in the blood, other body fluids, or tissues. A high level of biomarker may mean that a certain type of cancer is in the body. Examples of biomarkers include CA 125 (ovarian cancer), CA 15-3 (breast cancer), CEA (ovarian, lung, breast, pancreas, and gastrointestinal tract cancers), and PSA (prostate cancer). Also called tumor marker.

Biopsy (BY-op-see): The removal of cells or tissues for examination under a microscope. When only a sample of tissue is removed, the procedure is called an incisional biopsy or core biopsy. When an entire lump or suspicious area is removed, the procedure is called an excisional biopsy. When a sample of tissue or fluid is removed with a needle, the procedure is called a needle biopsy or fine-needle aspiration. Pleural biopsies are used to make the diagnosis of mesothelioma.

Biphasic: a mesothelioma which has both epithelial and sarcomatoid elements. Also called a mixed mesothelioma.

Bronchopleural fistula: a complication after extrapleural pneumonectomy in which there is a leakage of air from the closed bronchial tube.

C

Cachexia (ka-KEK-see-a): Loss of body weight and muscle mass, and weakness that may occur in patients with cancer, AIDS, or other chronic diseases. Cachexia is a common manifestation of late stage mesothelioma.

Cancer center: A hospital that specializes only in the care of patients with cancer. An NCI designated cancer center is specifically recognized and partially funded by the National Cancer Institute.

Cardiologist: a specialist in the treatment of conditions related to the heart who would perform the appropriate tests to see if a patient is functionally able to tolerate surgery for mesothelioma.

CAT scan: A series of detailed pictures of areas inside the body, taken from different angles; the pictures are created by a computer linked to an x-ray machine. Also called computerized axial tomography, computed tomography (CT scan), or computerized tomography.

Catheter: a tube which could be used to drain urine from the bladder; an intravenous catheter is used to give fluids in the vein.

Chemotherapy (kee-mo-THER-a-pee): Treatment with anticancer drugs. There are many varieties of these drugs which have different mechanisms for killing cancer cells.

Chest pain: Discomfort in the chest that can be a feeling of "heaviness" to a constant boring pain requiring narcotics.

Clinical trial: A type of research study that uses volunteers to test new methods of screening, prevention, diagnosis, or treatment of a disease. The trial may be carried out in a clinic or other medical facility. Also called a clinical study.

Cobalt machine: A radioactive machine using a form of the metal cobalt, which is used as a source of radiation to treat cancer.

Complementary and alternative medicine (CAM): Forms of treatment that are used in addition to (complementary) or instead of (alternative) standard treatments. These practices generally are not considered standard medical approaches. CAM may include dietary supplements, megadose vitamins, herbal preparations, special teas, acupuncture, massage therapy, magnet therapy, spiritual healing, and meditation.

Complete response: The disappearance of all signs of cancer in response to treatment. This does not always mean the cancer has been cured. Also called a complete remission.

Cytology: The study of cells using a microscope.

D

Diagnosis: The process of identifying a disease by the signs and symptoms.

Due diligence: The level of judgement, care, prudence, determination, and activity that a person would reasonably be expected to do under particular circumstances. It is a term used to imply in medicine that a patient has investigated the many options available for them after a diagnosis is made either by using second opinions or advice from the literature or other experts in order to make a decision about how and by whom he/she would like to be treated.

Dyspnea: Difficult, painful breathing or shortness of breath. One of the early symptoms of mesothelioma in the pleura due to the accumulation of fluid in the chest.

E

Echocardiogram: Echocardiogram is a test that uses sound waves to create a moving picture of the heart. The picture is much more detailed than X-ray image and involves no radiation exposure.

Empyema: infected fluid (pus) in the chest which can result postoperatively as a complication of surgery for mesothelioma.

EPA: The mission of the Environmental Protection Agency is to protect human health and the environment. It is particularly concerned with the protection of humans against cancer producing fibers like asbestos.

Epidural catheter: A catheter which allows injection of an anesthetic drug into the space between the wall of the spinal canal and the covering of the spinal cord. This is the most reliable means for short term pain relief after an operation for mesothelioma.

Epithelial (ep-ih-THEE-lee-ul): Refers to the cells that line the internal and external surfaces of the body and the term used to describe the appearance of the cells under the microscope for the most common type of mesothelioma.

Esophagitis: Inflammation of the esophagus (the tube that carries food from the mouth to the stomach). This most frequently occurs in the setting of chest radiation after operation for mesothelioma.

External-beam radiation (ray-dee-AY-shun): Radiation therapy that uses a machine to aim high-energy rays at the cancer. Also called external radiation. Most commonly used after removal of an entire lung for mesothelioma.

Extrapleural pneumonectomy: Surgery to remove a diseased lung, part of the pericardium (membrane covering the heart), part of the diaphragm (muscle between the lungs and the abdomen), and part of the parietal pleura (membrane lining the chest). This type of surgery is used most often to treat malignant mesothelioma.

F

Fibrosis: The growth of tissue containing or resembling fibers which can occur after radiation therapy or as scar after any disruption of normal tissue.

G

Gene therapy: Treatment that alters a gene. In studies of gene therapy for cancer, researchers are trying to improve the body's natural ability to fight the disease or to make the cancer cells more sensitive to other kinds of therapy by either adding a gene which was lost in the cancer or interfering with a gene which contributes to the growth of the cancer.

H

Health Maintenance Organization (HMO): A form of health insurance combining a range of coverages in a group basis. A group of doctors and other medical professionals offer care through the HMO for a flat monthly rate with no deductibles. However, only visits to professionals within the HMO network are covered by the policy. All visits, prescriptions and other care must be cleared by the HMO in order to be covered. A primary physician within the HMO handles referrals.

Heated chemoperfusion: The delivery of heated chemotherapy chemicals to the chest and/or abdomen in the operating room after the majority of the tumor is removed.

Hemoptysis: Coughing up blood.

Hemorrhage: In medicine, loss of blood from damaged blood vessels. A hemorrhage may be internal or external, and usually involves a lot of bleeding in a short time.

Hospice:

(HOS-pis): A program that provides special care for people who are near the end of life and for their families, either at home, in freestanding facilities, or within hospitals.

Hyperthermic or heated chemoperfusion: A procedure in which a warmed solution containing anticancer drugs is used to bathe, or is passed through the blood vessels of the tissue or organ containing the tumor.

I

Immunostaining: the use by pathologists of specific proteins with color producing labels attached to them to stain tissue sections in order to differentiate one tumor from another. Particularly important to use a battery of immunostains in order to tell whether the biopsy is a mesothelioma or a lung cancer.

Informed consent: A process in which a person learns key facts about a clinical trial, including potential risks and benefits, before deciding whether or not to participate in a study. Informed consent continues throughout the trial.

Intensity-modulated radiation therapy (IMRT): A type of 3-dimensional radiation therapy that uses computer-generated images to show the size and shape of the tumor. Thin beams of radiation of different intensities are aimed at the tumor from many angles. This type of radiation therapy reduces the damage to healthy tissue near the tumor and is being explored in mesothelioma in order to treat only the involved pleural and spare normal tissue.

Intravenous (in-tra-VEE-nus) (IV): Within a blood vessel.

Invasive cancer: Cancer that has spread beyond the layer of tissue in which it developed and is growing into surrounding, healthy tissues. Also called infiltrating cancer.

L

Latency period: The time between the actual exposure to a carcinogen like asbestos and the development of cancer, i.e. mesothelioma.

Linear accelerator: A machine that creates high-energy radiation to treat cancer, using electricity to form a stream of fast-moving subatomic particles. Also called mega-voltage (MeV) linear accelerator or a linac.

Local anesthetic: the use of an injectable drug in the area of a biopsy to deaden the area.

Local recurrence: reappearance of the previously treated cancer at its original site; with mesothelioma, a local recurrence occurs in the pleura most frequently after surgery for the tumor.

Lymph: Fluid composed of lymphocytes.

Lymphatic vessels: Interconnecting tubes that link lymph nodes and allow flow of lymph.

Lymph node (limf node): A rounded mass of lymphatic tissue that is surrounded by a capsule of connective tissue. Lymph nodes filter lymph (lymphatic fluid), and they store lymphocytes (white blood cells). They are located along lymphatic vessels.

Also called a lymph gland. The involvement of lymph glands by mesothelioma changes the stage to a higher one and is an indication of a more advanced tumor.

Lymphocyte (LIM-fo-site): A type of white blood cell. Lymphocytes have a number of roles in the immune system, including the production of antibodies and other substances that fight infection and diseases.

M

Magnetic resonance imaging (mag-NET-ik REZ-o-nans IM-a-jing) (MRI): A procedure in which radio waves and a powerful magnet linked to a computer are used to create detailed pictures of areas inside the body. These pictures can show the difference between normal and diseased tissue. MRI makes better images of organs and soft tissue than other scanning techniques, such as CT or x-ray. MRI is especially useful for imaging the brain, spine, the soft tissue of joints, and the inside of bones. Also called nuclear magnetic resonance imaging.

Malignant seeding: growth of a tumor at a site which may be outside its original domain because of contamination of a new site with malignant cells after a biopsy or from cells in a malignant effusion.

Mediastinoscopy (MEE-dee-a-stin-AHS-ko-pee): A procedure in which a tube is inserted into the chest to view the organs in the area between the lungs and nearby lymph nodes. The tube is inserted through an incision above the breastbone. This procedure is usually performed to get a tissue sample from the lymph nodes on the right side of the chest.

Medical oncologist: A specially certified physician who treats cancer and delivers chemotherapy.

Metastasis (meh-TAS-ta-sis): The spread of cancer from one part of the body to another. A tumor formed by cells that have spread is called a "metastatic tumor" or a "metastasis." The metastatic tumor contains cells that are like those in the original (primary) tumor. The plural form of metastasis is metastases (meh-TAS-ta-seez).

Metastatic recurrence: Return of the cancer at a site away from the original site.

Molecularly targeted therapy: In cancer treatment, substances that kill cancer cells by targeting key molecules involved in cancer cell growth.

Multimodality treatment: Therapy that combines more than one method of treatment.

N

Narcotic: An agent that causes insensibility or stupor; usually refers to opioids given to relieve pain.

Neuropathy: A problem in peripheral nerve function (any part of the nervous system except the brain and spinal cord) that causes pain, numbness, tingling, swelling, and muscle weakness in various parts of the body. Neuropathies may be caused by physical injury, infection, toxic substances, disease (e.g., cancer, diabetes, kidney failure, or malnutrition), or drugs such as anticancer drugs. Also called peripheral neuropathy.

O

Oncology: The study of cancer.

OSHA: the Occupational and Safety Health Administration is a government agency which regulates the use of asbestos and sets the standards for its distribution.

P

Paracentesis: Insertion of a thin needle or tube into the abdomen to remove fluid from the peritoneal cavity. Commonly used to make the diagnosis of peritoneal mesothelioma in patients with ascites or to diagnose recurrence of the disease in the belly.

Parietal pleura: the lining on the inside of the chest wall which is composed of mesothelial cells and is the target organ for asbestos induced mesothelioma.

Partial response: A decrease in the size of a tumor, or in the extent of cancer in the body, in response to treatment.

Pathologist (pa-THOL-o-jist): A doctor who identifies diseases by studying cells and tissues under a microscope.

Peptide: Any compound consisting of two or more amino acids, the building blocks of proteins.

Performance status: A measure of how well a patient is able to perform ordinary tasks and carry out daily activities.

Pericardium: the heart sac that covers the heart.

Peritoneoscopy: The use of a think lighted tube (called a laparoscope to examine the abdomen).

Peritoneum (PAIR-ih-toc-NEE-um): The tissue that lines the abdominal wall and covers most of the organs in the abdomen which is composed of mesothelial cells and is the target organ for abdominal mesothelioma.

PET scan: Positron emission tomography scan. A procedure in which a small amount of radioactive glucose (sugar) is injected into a vein, and a scanner is used to make detailed, computerized pictures of areas inside the body where the glucose is used. Because cancer cells often use more glucose than normal cells, the pictures can be used to find cancer cells in the body.

Photodynamic therapy (foe-toe-dye-NAM-ik): Treatment with drugs that become active when exposed to light. These drugs kill cancer cells.

Platelet (PLAYT-let): A type of blood cell that helps prevent bleeding by causing blood clots to form. Also called a thrombocyte.

Pleura (PLOOR-a): A thin layer of tissue covering the lungs and lining the interior wall of the chest cavity. It protects and cushions the lungs. This tissue secretes a small amount of fluid that acts as a lubricant, allowing the lungs to move smoothly in the chest cavity while breathing.

Pleural cavity: The space enclosed by the pleura, which is a thin layer of tissue that covers the lungs and lines the interior wall of the chest cavity.

Pleural effusion: An abnormal collection of fluid between the thin layers of tissue (pleura) lining the lung and the wall of the chest cavity.

Pleurectomy/decortication: an operation for mesothelioma that removes the involved pleura and frees the underlying lung so that it can expand and fill the pleural cavity.

Pleurodesis (PLOO-ro-DEE-sis): A medical procedure that uses chemicals or drugs to cause inflammation and adhesion between the layers of the pleura (the tissue that covers the lungs and lines the interior wall of the chest cavity). This prevents the buildup of fluid in the pleural cavity. It is used as a treatment for severe pleural effusion. Can be performed with a variety of agents.

Pneumonectomy (noo-mo-NEK-toe-mee): An operation to remove an entire lung.

Pneumonitis (noo-MONE-ya): An inflammatory infection that occurs in the lung.

Pneumothorax: air within the chest cavity.

Prognosis (prog-NO-sis): The likely outcome or course of a disease; the chance of recovery or recurrence.

Progressive disease: Cancer that is increasing in scope or severity.

Protein (PRO-teen): A molecule made up of amino acids that are needed for the body to function properly. Proteins are the basis of body structures such as skin and hair and of substances such as enzymes, cytokines, and antibodies.

Protocol: An action plan for a clinical trial. The plan states what the study will do, how, and why. It explains how many people will be in it, who is eligible to participate, what study agents or other interventions they will be given, what tests they will receive and how often, and what information will be gathered.

Pulmonary embolism: migration of a clot, usually from the legs, to the heart resulting in the blockage of arteries to the lung and resulting in acute shortness of breath. A possible cause of morbidity and mortality from operations for mesothelioma.

Pulmonary function test: a series of breathing maneuvers performed in a certified laboratory which measures the capacity of the lungs and the force with which an individual can inhale and exhale.

Q

Quantititative lung perfusion scan: a radioactive nuclear scan which allows the measurement of the function of individual lung segments which can be used to determine how an individual will tolerate loss of lung function for an operation for mesothelioma.

R

Radiation (ray-dee-AY-shun): Energy released in the form of particles or electromagnetic waves. Common sources of radiation include radon gas, cosmic rays from outer space, and medical x-rays.

Radiation oncologist: a physician who delivers radiation.

Radiology: The use of radiation (such as x-rays) or other imaging technologies (such as ultrasound and magnetic resonance imaging) to diagnose or treat disease.

Recurrence: The return of cancer, at the same site as the original (primary) tumor or in another location, after the tumor had disappeared.

Recurrent cancer: Cancer that has returned after a period of time during which the cancer could not be detected. The cancer may come back to the same site as the original (primary) tumor or to another place in the body.

Red blood cell: A cell that carries oxygen to all parts of the body. Also called an erythrocyte.

Referral: A primary physician seeks expert consultation in cases by referring the patient to a specialist who may or may not be associated with a cancer center.

Regional recurrence: Return of the cancer in a location close to the original cancer.

Remission: A decrease in or disappearance of signs and symptoms of cancer. In partial remission, some, but not all, signs and symptoms of cancer have disappeared. In complete remission, all signs and symptoms of cancer have disappeared, although cancer still may be in the body.

Response: The results measured either by x-ray or physical exam of treatment that compares the status (usually the size) of the tumor before treatment to its status after treatment.

S

Sarcomatoid: the least common variant of mesothelioma which has the appearance under the microscope of spindly cells which look like supportive or connective tissue.

Stable disease: Cancer that is neither decreasing nor increasing in extent or severity.

Staging (STAY-jing): Performing exams and tests to learn the extent of the cancer within the body, especially whether the disease has spread from the original site to other parts of the body. It is important to know the stage of the disease in order to plan the best treatment.

Standard of care: In medicine, treatment that experts agree is appropriate, accepted, and widely used. Health care providers are obligated to provide patients with the standard of care. Also called standard therapy or best practice.

Standard therapy: In medicine, treatment that experts agree is appropriate, accepted, and widely used. Health care providers are obligated to provide patients with standard therapy. Also called standard of care or best practice.

Supportive care: Care given to improve the quality of life of patients who have a serious or life-threatening disease. The goal of supportive care is to prevent or treat as early as possible the symptoms of the disease, side effects caused by treatment of the disease, and psychological, social, and spiritual problems related to the disease or its treatment. Also called palliative care, comfort care, and symptom management.

T

Thoracentesis (thor-a-sen-TEE-sis): Removal of fluid from the pleural cavity through a needle inserted between the ribs.

Thoracic (thor-ASS-ik): Having to do with the chest.

Thoracic surgical oncologist: A general thoracic surgeon whose practice is almost exclusively the treatment of cancers in the chest and who does not perform heart surgery.

Thoracoscopy: The use of a thin, lighted tube (called an endoscope) to examine the inside of the chest.

Thoracotomy (thor-a-KAH-toe-mee): An operation to open the chest.

Toxic: Having to do with poison or something harmful to the body. Toxic substances usually cause unwanted side effects.

V

Visceral pleura: the mesothelial lining on the surface of the lung which can also be a target organ for mesothelioma.

W

White blood cell (WBC): Refers to a blood cell that does not contain hemoglobin. White blood cells include lymphocytes, neutrophils, eosinophils, macrophages, and mast cells. These cells are made by bone marrow and help the body fight infection and other diseases.

Workup: A series of tests to discover information about the patient, most commonly to define extent of disease or suitability for a given treatment.

Index